Atlas for the
Diagnosis of Tumors
in the Dog and Cat

Atlas for the Diagnosis of Tumors in the Dog and Cat

Anita R. Kiehl, DVM, MS, Diplomate ACVP

Maron Brown Calderwood Mays, VMD, PhD, Diplomate ACVP

WILEY Blackwell

Library of Congress Cataloging-in-Publication Data

Names: Kiehl, Anita R., author. | Calderwood Mays, Maron B., author.
Title: Atlas for the diagnosis of tumors in the dog and cat / Anita R. Kiehl, Maron Brown Calderwood Mays.
Description: Ames, Iowa : John Wiley and Sons, Inc., 2016. | Includes bibliographical references and index.
Identifiers: LCCN 2016014281 (print) | LCCN 2016015089 (ebook) | ISBN 9781119051213 (cloth) |
    ISBN 9781119051152 (pdf) | ISBN 9781119050797 (epub)
Subjects: | MESH: Neoplasms–veterinary | Neoplasms–diagnosis | Neoplasms–pathology |
    Prognosis | Dog Diseases | Cat Diseases | Atlases
Classification: LCC SF910.T8 (print) | LCC SF910.T8 (ebook) | NLM SF 910.T8 | DDC 636.089/6994–dc23
LC record available at http://lccn.loc.gov/2016014281

A catalogue record for this book is available from the British Library.

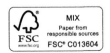

This work was inspired by the veterinary practitioners who give so much effort to caring for the pets that are an integral part of loving families and the many future pets seeking a family.

Contents

Preface

Practitioners of the healing arts are trained to understand how the body functions as a community of organ systems that operates cooperatively in healthy homeostasis, and how they may lose varying degrees of function due to infectious, traumatic, or mechanical injury. In many cases it is not an "all or nothing" situation.

A diagnosis or even a suspicion of cancer sometimes elicits a different reaction, evoking a black versus white, "either you have cancer or you don't" response. The discovery of a mass can lead to an immediate and unsubstantiated assumption of fatal disease. This can delay evaluation and treatment of lesions that could be mitigated or cured if addressed in an early time frame.

The first chapter of this atlas is intended to give a brief overview of the methods used to produce a diagnosis and prognosis from a biopsy tissue sample. In the subsequent chapters, light microscope-derived pictures of biopsy samples are paired with photomicrographs of cells obtained via fine needle aspiration (FNA), and certain signature findings applicable to both methods are compared as a means to bring additional point of care tools to the diagnostic menu.

The final chapter discusses sample handling, staining, and shipping, and although it is presented at the end of the text, achievement of a useful diagnosis really starts here.

Acknowledgments

Anita R. Kiehl DVM, MS, DACVP

I would like to thank my family: Arland, Nick, Isabelle, and Marlon, for their encouragement and support. I would like to thank my friends Drs. Laura Hockett, Rachel Hill, and Jim Benson for their inspiration and for their help with my renewed journey in clinical medicine. I would like to thank Drs. Rose Manducca, Karen Trainor, and Rachel Hill for proofing, editing, and moral support, and Susan Shipp for manuscript support. I am grateful for the excellent histology slides produced by National Biovet Lab and Northwest Arkansas Pathology. Last but not least I thank the staff at Florida Vet Path, especially Lacie Laielli, for their organizing assistance and office support.

Maron Brown Calderwood Mays VMD, PhD, DACVP

Thank you Dr. David Mays, my patient husband, for his experienced editorial advice and his periodic help with large gross specimens that require the use of my band saw. Also, thank you Histology Tech Services, Inc., Gainesville, FL—Beverly and Doug Robinson and Andrew Brown—for the careful specimen trimming, the flawless glass histology slides, and their expertise with myriad special stains that make it possible for me to do my job each day. I also thank my transcriptionists, Analee McLain, Susan Allee, and Vicky Baldwin, for their attention to detail, accuracy, and quick turnaround, and for their help in developing our huge veterinary pathology Spell Check dictionary. In addition, I thank my courier, Gloria Neff, who picks up and delivers samples and slides efficiently all over north-central Florida five days a week for Florida Vet Path, Inc. Thanks to our office staff who keep track of all the samples and reports, and answer numerous questions from clients daily. Finally, thanks to our clients, the conscientious veterinarians in clinical practice who faithfully send us their samples with detailed clinical histories, and often with clinical follow-up. This atlas would not have been possible without all of these wonderful people.

PART I

Overview of the Diagnostic Process

1   Overview of Grading and Staging

Identification of the process

Tumor is a word of Latin derivation meaning a swelling or protruberance—a "mass." In its broadest sense it includes masses formed by cellular inflammatory infiltrates, controlled proliferations of hyperplastic cells, and uncontrolled proliferations of neoplastic cells (cancer). Controlled proliferations of cells have a recognizable structure, may perform their usual physiologic function, do not invade local tissues, and suffer senescence and programmed cell death (apoptosis). Uncontrolled proliferations may contain cells of variable structure, may be functional or nonfunctional, may invade local tissues or cause local tissue necrosis by their increasing bulk, replicate in a disorderly manner, and do not suffer programmed cell death.

The path to successful treatment of a tumor begins with recognition of the lesion on a gross level, usually by the caretaker of a dog or cat, sometimes by a groomer, or often during a physical exam by a veterinarian. The next step is assignment of the pathological process into a category of inflammation, hyperplasia, or neoplasia, or some combination of these categories. This can be accomplished at the point of care by aspirating the lesion with a needle and examining the individual cells. In the following chapters this will be called fine needle aspiration (FNA). With some tumors, especially papillomas, impression or scraping of the lesion can yield diagnostic cells, but generally this is not the ideal method of collection, as surface contamination can make evaluation difficult. All cytologic samples are stained with Wright-Giemsa (W-G) stain unless otherwise indicated.

Figure 1.1 shows an apocrine gland adenoma FNA. This cluster of small epithelial cells is suggestive of a proliferation of basaloid epithelial cells or the ductular epithelium of an apocrine gland. The cell nuclei are small and regular, and there is scant inflammation, as shown by the neutrophil in this field.

When FNA of a mass reveals a population of proliferating cells, indicating the lesion is not merely an influx of inflammatory cells that can be relieved by medical means, biopsy allows histopathological evaluation of the affected tissue, showing the architectural arrangement of the cells and allowing for a more definitive diagnosis. This is the point where a hyperplastic growth is distinguished from a neoplastic growth based on how the cells are structurally arranged. FNA cannot evaluate architectural arrangement accurately, because the cells are usually stripped of their association by the process of aspiration. The decision to take an incisional biopsy that removes a portion of the mass, or an excisional biopsy that removes all of the mass, should be based on factors such as the tumor type suggested by the FNA, the size of the lesion, the location of the lesion, the stage of the disease, and other parameters such as the overall health of the patient and wishes of the owner. Ultimately the decision rests on the clinical judgment of the surgeon. All biopsies shown in the following pages are stained with hematoxalin and eosin (H&E), unless otherwise indicated.

Figure 1.2 is a biopsy showing the architecture of the gland aspirated in Figure 1.1. There are double rows of small epithelial cells proliferating in a manner that does not invade into the adjacent stroma, indicating that this is a benign apocrine gland tumor referred to as an apocrine ductular adenoma.

FNA can sometimes identify cells that are so clearly abnormal, either by morphology or cell density, that neoplasia can be diagnosed on a presumptive basis.

Figure 1.3 shows a transitional cell carcinoma FNA. An adult female mixed breed dog was presented for hematuria and dysuria. A tentative diagnosis of cystitis was made based on clinical signs, and cystocentesis was performed to collect urine for routine urinalysis and sedimentation. Cytologic exam revealed many clusters of large epithelioid cells with

Atlas for the Diagnosis of Tumors in the Dog and Cat, First Edition. Anita R. Kiehl and Maron Brown Calderwood Mays.
© 2016 John Wiley & Sons, Inc. Published 2016 by John Wiley & Sons, Inc.

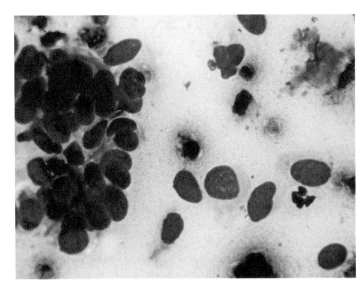

Figure 1.1 Apocrine gland adenoma FNA. 50x.

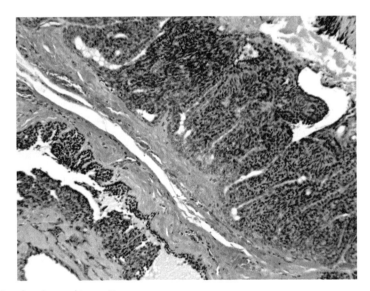

Figure 1.2 Apocrine gland ductular adenoma biopsy. 40x.

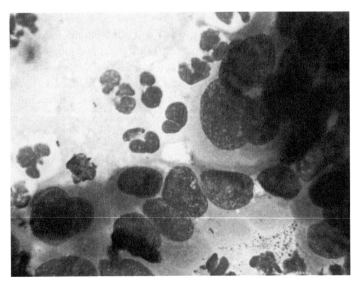

Figure 1.3 Transitional cell carcinoma FNA. 50x.

marked anisokaryosis (variation in nuclear size) and basophilic cytoplasm. There were scattered neutrophils, erythrocytes, and cellular debris. No infectious agents were seen. A preliminary diagnosis of neoplasia, probable transitional cell carcinoma, was made. Treatment for infectious cystitis, based just on clinical signs, would prove useless and would delay the true diagnosis. If neoplasia is suspected on presentation, catheterization would be the preferable method of collection.

If biopsy identifies the process as hyperplastic, and the margins are free of abnormal cells, it can be assumed that the lesion is cured. This does not preclude additional lesions arising adjacent to the removed mass.

If biopsy identifies the process as neoplastic, the tumor can be categorized into type and grade based on published guidelines derived from scores of biopsies and the statistical analysis of their behavior. The purpose of this atlas is to enable visual recognition of lesions and thus the reader will be spared a detailed description of the original research that forms the basis for statistical analysis. Inquiring minds, however, are encouraged to review the documents in the additional journals and books listed in the reference section.

Identification of tumor types

The broadest categories of tumor types are derived from tissue of origin. Epithelial origin tumors are designated as epithelioma or adenoma (benign) and carcinoma (malignant). Mesenchymal origin tumors are typically designated as an –oma prefixed by the tissue of origin (benign) or -sarcoma prefixed by the tissue of origin (malignant). Discrete cells lacking cell to cell adhesion and originating from the specialized tissue and circulating cells of the immune system, such as lymphocytes, plasma cells, histiocytes, mast cells, and a transplantable chymeric neoplasm called transmissible venereal tumor, are designated as round cell tumors, often –omas, prefixed by the tissue of origin (and indicated as benign or malignant). There is a separate category for melanoma, which can have epithelioid, spindloid, and round cell characteristics within the same tumor (both benign and malignant).

Grading

Grading is performed by the pathologist using parameters that can only be assessed by biopsy, including mitotic activity per high power (40x) field, the presence of a recognizable pattern of growth, and invasion into adjacent normal tissue. Mitotic activity is an important part of most grading systems. Mitotic rate or mitotic count is the number of mitotic figures per high-power field (mitotic figures/HPF).[1] Mitotic index (MI) is generally accepted as the number of mitotic figures in 10 fields (mitotic figures/10 HPF), but if a different number of fields have been used, it must be stated in the numerical figure.[2] Both mitotic rate and mitotic index can vary widely depending on which areas of the tumor are examined. The presence of necrosis and dense inflammatory infiltrates can make identification of mitotic figures difficult, and small biopsies less than 10 fields in size can make enumeration of the mitotic index impossible. Thus, grade is not based just on mitotic activity but also on other aspects of the proliferating population such as the amount of necrosis (also subjective and based on the section examined) and pattern of growth in the tissue. This heterogeneity introduces some variation into the assessment of tumor grade and has contributed to the proliferation of several grading systems for some tumors as pathologists attempt to find the best system (Table 1.1).

Grading systems can use a quantifiable descriptive term such as low, medium, and high grade or can assign a numerical label (Table 1.2), and grading systems can use an equation to score several critical features that add up to a sum assigned to a grade (Table 1.3). All of the systems used are designed to succinctly convey the probability that a tumor will be aggressive and likely to invade local or distant tissues. Grading also allows a pathologist to give an oncologist a specified set of details designed to help choose and monitor appropriate therapy. The general practitioner and the oncologist or internist may have different preferences for grading protocols or treatment plans, and may desire

Table 1.1 Multiple grading systems for lymphoma.

Tumor	System	Features
Lymphoma	NCI WF	pattern, biology, survival
	Kiel	pattern, morphology, immunophenotype
	WHO	pattern, morphology, immunophenotype

Table 1.2 Multiple grading systems for mast cell tumor.

Tumor	System, reference	Grade; features
MCT	Patnaik, 1.27	1; confined to dermis, 0 mitoses/HPF, uniform nuclei 2; invades subcutis, 0–1 mitoses/hpf, rare binucleate cells 3; invades deep tissues, >3 mitoses in some fields, pleomorphic nuclei
	MSU, 1.28	low; rare mitoses, confined to dermis, uniform nuclei high; invasive, frequent mitoses, pleomorphic nuclei

Table 1.3 Grading systems based on points for sarcoma in canines and mammary gland tumor in canines.

Tumor	Reference	Features
Sarcoma	1.20	Differentiation 1; regular appearance 2; poorly differentiated 3; pleomorphic Mitoses 1;0–9 2; 10–19 2; 10–19 Tumor necrosis 1; no necrosis 2; <50% necrosis 3; >50% necrosis Score 1; 3 or less 2; 4–5 3; 6 or more
Mammary tumor	1.14	Tubule formation: 1; >75% 2; 10–75% 3; <10% Nuclear form: 1; uniform 2; variation 3; pleomorphic Mitoses/10 HPS 1; 0–9/10 HPF 2; 10–19/10 HPF 3; 20+/10 HPF Score: 1; low, 3–5 2; moderate, 6–7 3; high, 8–9

different sets of information, resulting in a report listing several grading protocols applicable to the tumor described. These compilations of data can be useful even in the face of periodic modification as the database grows and our diagnostic tools become more refined to include molecular diagnostic parameters such as tumor growth fraction, genetic analysis for c-KIT gene mutation which activates the KIT tyrosine kinase receptor, and polymerase chain reaction (PCR) of antigen receptor site rearrangements. Open communication between clinicians and specialists will be necessary to keep apprised of new developments.

Figure 1.4 shows a squamous cell carcinoma (SCC) biopsy with two mitotic figures. The cells in this biopsy are fairly well differentiated and recognizable as squamous epithelial cells and the mitotic figures (arrows) are clear.

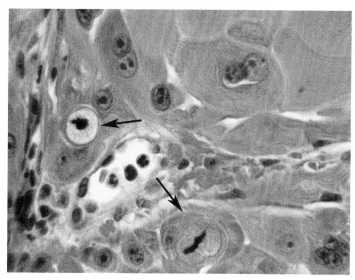

Figure 1.4 Squamous cell carcinoma biopsy. 50x.

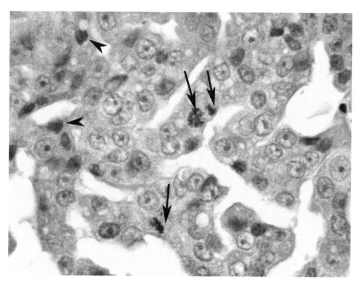

Figure 1.5 Apocrine adenocarcinoma biopsy. 50x.

Evaluation of at least 10 high power (40x) fields is recommended for assigning a grade. Fragmented or crushed tissue and biopsies smaller than 1.0 centimeter (cm) may have insufficient fields for proper evaluation of mitotic index.

Figure 1.5 shows an apocrine adenocarcinoma biopsy with three definitive (arrows) and two questionable (arrowheads) mitotic figures. Cells with vague and pyknotic nuclei can be difficult to assess for mitotic activity, a situation that introduces a source of discrepancy in the grading of some tumors. Necrosis and inflammation compound the problem by increasing the number of active and dying cells that are not necessarily tumor cells. Evaluation of 10 fields can be impossible if only tiny fragments are submitted for biopsy.

Staging

Staging is a clinical assessment and quantifies information such as the location of the tumor in the body, the size of the tumor, and whether there is local lymphatic or distant metastasis. The clinician must perform staging, but the pathologist can be of assistance if adjacent stroma or lymphatic tissue is submitted for analysis and lymphatic or vascular invasion can be documented on biopsy tissues.

Figure 1.6 shows lymphatic metastasis of mammary carcinoma. This biopsy of a mammary carcinoma revealed dilated lymphatics containing invasive carcinoma cells. This will only be seen if adjacent normal tissue containing lymphatics is included in the biopsy sample. Often the best area to look for compromised lymphatics is the subepidermis, therefore, it is helpful to submit the skin over the mass and at lateral margins, as well as deeper tissue.

Figure 1.7 shows lymph node metastasis of mammary carcinoma. This biopsy of a mammary tumor included a local lymph node that was found to have invasive carcinoma. This is where the pathologist can be helpful in the staging process.

There are some factors that can affect the use of grade and stage. Grade and stage are dynamic, not static, and each can progress independently to a different level. Grade and stage have elements of subjectivity; grade is based on a thin section of only a portion of the affected tissue so sampling error is not impossible, while stage can be affected by the quality and type of diagnostic procedures used (such as radiography versus magnetic resonance imaging). If grade and stage are used to predict future behavior, the classification systems must have a sound basis and be applicable to the species and disease process to which they applied. Histiocytic proliferations are infamous for their ability to regress or progress, spread to multiple sites, or completely disappear in dogs, yet they are, as currently recognized, always progressively more aggressive in cats.[3] It is important to recognize species and maybe even breed variability in behavior.

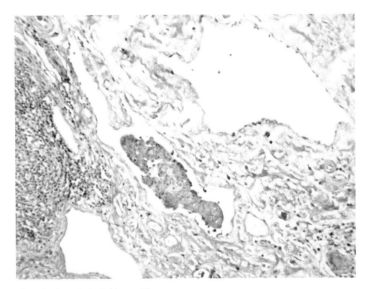

Figure 1.6 Mammary carcinoma lymphatic metastasis biopsy. 20x.

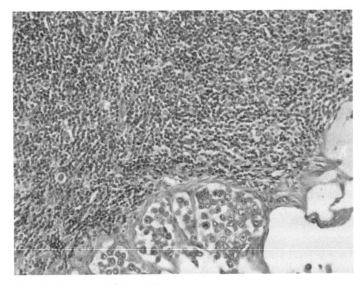

Figure 1.7 Mammary carcinoma lymph node metastasis biopsy. 10x.

Mast cell tumors in Siamese cats will sometimes spontaneously regress, but this would not be expected in Domestic Shorthair breeds (nor in dogs of any breed). Some tumors vary in behavior by site of origin and may have differing staging systems depending on location. Additionally, in some studies of melanocytic and mammary tumors the presence of neoplastic cells in local lymphatics may not be correlated with survival time.[4, 5] The database is constantly expanding, and consultation with a specialist can provide the most current recommendations.

Staging versus clinical behavior

A patient that presents with multiple masses can have a wide range of outcomes dependent on the type of process causing the masses. A multifocal infectious or inflammatory disease might be expected to have a better prognosis than a widespread neoplastic disease. Aspiration of multiple masses is recommended as a first step because this will help determine if the masses are due to one process or multiple etiologies and can indicate infectious versus neoplastic etiology. This approach can yield the most favorable clinical outcome by treating the correct disease without delay. Staging will only be applicable after the disease process has been definitively diagnosed, regardless of how widespread the disease appears clinically.

Figure 1.8 shows a fungal granuloma. An adult male neutered cat presented with multiple skin masses, and aspiration of several masses revealed scattered histiocytes, small lymphocytes, macrophages, and *Cryptococcus neoformans*. The presence of a fungal agent indicates antifungal medical therapy would be appropriate, but immunosuppressive drugs or chemotherapy agents would be contraindicated and antibacterial therapy would be ineffective. The diagnosis made by FNA allows for timely therapy prior to biopsy in this case.

Figure 1.9 shows a *Cryptococcus neoformans* biopsy. This adult male neutered cat had multiple skin masses about the head and in the submandibular area, aspirates of which are illustrated in Figure 1.8. The nodules persisted despite therapy, and biopsy revealed *Cryptococcus* organisms both in the skin nodules and lymph nodes. This disease may progress even with appropriate medical therapy, and this neurotropic organism can infiltrate the tissues of the nasal cavity, spreading to local lymph nodes and eventually invading the brain. Testing for immunosuppressive virus infection would be prudent.

Figure 1.10 shows a canine histiocytoma. Aspirate of several cutaneous masses in this 2-year-old dog revealed many round cells with fine chromatin and pale cytoplasm as well as scattered small lymphocytes and neutrophils. The preliminary diagnosis was multifocal histiocytoma, and biopsy was recommended for definitive diagnosis because the lesions were multiple and persistent. Biopsy is not usually indicated at first presentation of this tumor type if there is only one mass and it regresses in a timely manner.

Figure 1.11 shows a canine cutaneous histiocytoma. This biopsy revealed that recurrent skin masses in a young dog were composed of sheets of round cells with moderate pale cytoplasm, occasional mitotic figures, and rare invasion into the epithelial layer by solitary cells. This lesion is expected to regress with time. If this mass fails to regress,

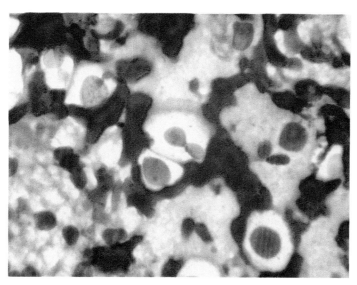

Figure 1.8 Fungal granuloma FNA. 50x.

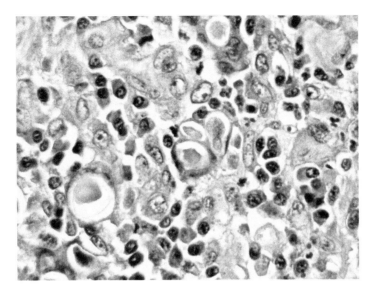

Figure 1.9 *Cryptococcus neoformans* biopsy. 40x.

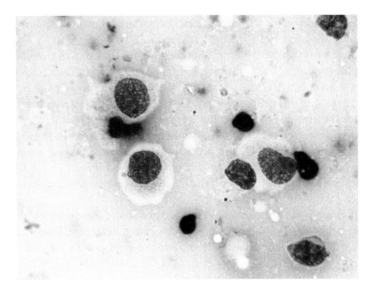

Figure 1.10 Canine histiocytoma FNA. 50x.

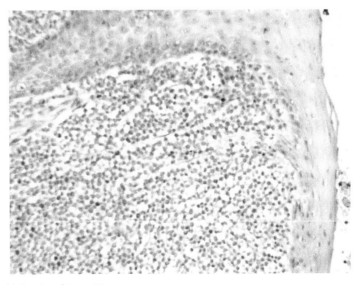

Figure 1.11 Canine cutaneous histiocytoma biopsy. 10x.

additional slides could be cut from the same block of fixed tissue used for the H&E slide and evaluated with Giemsa stain to exclude poorly granular mast cell tumor. Immunohistochemical markers for T and B lymphocytes could also be applied to additional freshly cut slides to exclude cutaneous lymphoma. If there are concomitant genital masses, transmissible venereal tumor should be considered. Additional immunohistochemical markers for histiocytes and other cell types are also available and are usually performed at research centers for best results. Consultation with laboratory personnel, the diagnostic pathologist that will be reading the tissue, and referral specialists such as oncologists or internists who may be working on the case, will often yield the best plan for additional special stains in cases of persistent or progressive histiocytic tumors.

Figure 1.12 shows a cutaneous lymphoma via FNA. Aspirate of multiple skin masses on an adult, spayed female mixed breed dog yielded a dense population of monomorphic round cells, about the size of the accompanying neutrophil, with round to occasionally cleaved nuclei, slightly clumped chromatin, and scant lightly basophilic cytoplasm. The preliminary diagnosis is cutaneous lymphoma.

Figure 1.13 shows a cutaneous lymphoma biopsy. Biopsy of several skin masses on the trunk of the adult dog in Figure 1.12 revealed variably dense infiltrates of fairly monomorphic medium-sized round cells that are invading into the epidermis and forming microabscesses. This epithelial invasion is a hallmark of epitheliotrophic cutaneous T-cell lymphoma. Unlike the histiocytoma in the previous figure, this disease will be progressive, and early therapy is usually indicated. If this is an indolent T-cell lymphoma, the rate of progression may be slow in the early stages.[6]

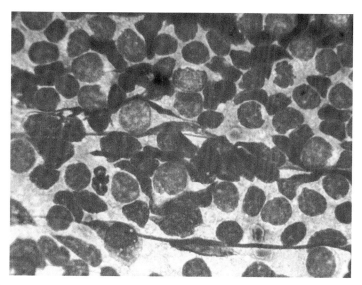

Figure 1.12 Cutaneous lymphoma FNA. 50x.

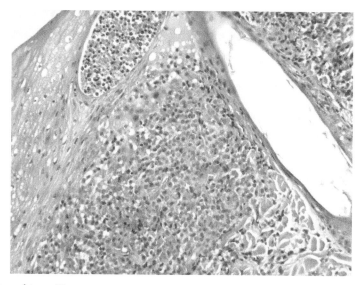

Figure 1.13 Cutaneous lymphoma biopsy. 20x.

These three disease processes can have a somewhat similar clinical appearance but have distinguishing cytologic and histologic features that allow accurate diagnosis and therefore a more applicable prognosis and therapeutic regimen. Multiple skin masses and lymphadenopathy have different significance in these three diseases and therefore any staging or prognostic categorization must be done with a definitive diagnosis in hand.

Epithelial tumors

Epithelial neoplasms can arise as benign (epithelioma, adenoma) or malignant (carcinoma) tumors. Benign tumors may undergo transformation to malignant tumors.

Figure 1.14 shows an apocrine gland adenoma biopsy. This skin mass is composed of cystic spaces lined by single to double rows of well-differentiated apocrine epithelium, consisting of cells with small nuclei and scant cytoplasm that do not invade into underlying stroma. This tumor is benign, and complete excision with conservative margins of 0.2 cm should be curative.

Figure 1.15 shows an apocrine gland carcinoma biopsy. This invasive tumor can arise from an apocrine gland in the skin and rapidly invade adjacent stroma and lymphatic structures. There may be remnants of glands filled with

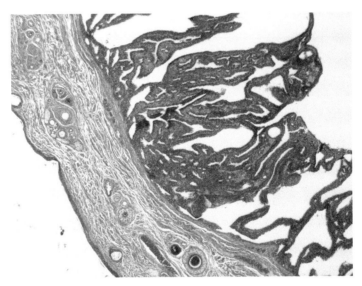

Figure 1.14 Apocrine gland adenoma biopsy. 10x.

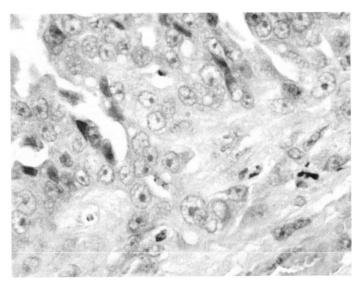

Figure 1.15 Apocrine gland carcinoma biopsy. 40x.

neoplastic cells, or the cells may form sheets in the stroma with only a suggestion of the former glandular architecture. The nuclei are large with large nucleoli and vesiculated chromatin. There is cellular disorganization even in areas of retained glandular structure. Local lymph nodes and thoracic radiographs should be evaluated for evidence of metastasis. Complete, wide excision is the minimal approach, and continued monitoring for regrowth or evidence of metastasis is advisable. Consultation with an oncologist would be helpful to determine the current most efficacious approach for medical therapy.

Mammary chains are exposed to systemic factors known to promote mammary neoplasia, and therefore, it is not unusual for dogs and cats to experience tumors in multiple glands, and multiple tumors of the same or different type in the same gland. It is well established that in the mammary gland hyperplastic lesions and benign tumors can develop into malignant tumors if not removed early or if incompletely removed.[7]

Figure 1.16 shows a complex mammary adenoma biopsy with focal transformation to ductular carcinoma in an adjacent lobule. The larger mass in the lower right quadrant (arrow) is a complex, low-grade mammary tumor, which is not invading into surrounding stroma. In the upper center of the slide there is a proliferation of ducts/alveoli (arrowhead) exhibiting focal atypia characterized by filling of the ducts with moderately pleomorphic epithelial cells that appear to have lost the normal arrangement of basally located nuclei that defines the normal duct. This demonstrates, at light microscope level, the concept of how plump, presumably hyperplastic cells might undergo loss of normal regulatory control, filling the ducts with disorganized epithelial cells and eventually escaping into the surrounding stroma.

Figure 1.17 shows a closer view of the developing carcinoma in Figure 1.16. There is an irregular proliferation of cells filling rather than lining the tubules and exhibiting larger than normal nuclei with open chromatin, a probable mitotic

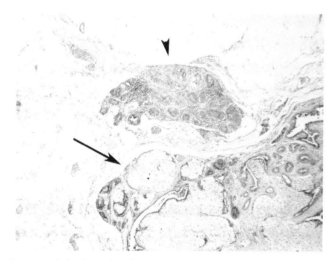

Figure 1.16 Complex mammary adenoma with focal intraductal carcinoma biopsy. 10x.

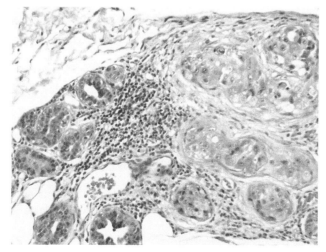

Figure 1.17 Mammary intraductular carcinoma. 40x.

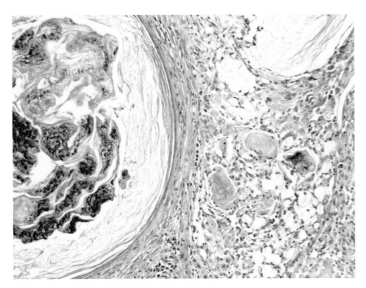

Figure 1.18 Trichoepithelioma biopsy. 20x.

figure, and abundant more deeply basophilic cytoplasm than the cells in the adjacent tubules. There appears to be early peritubular fibrosis and a peritubular inflammatory infiltrate of small lymphocytes and plasma cells. A more aggressive mammary tumor appears to be arising within this lobule. There is a recognizable inflammatory infiltrate of small lymphocytes and plasma cells associated with this lesion.

Epithelial tumors can arise from the many structures of the haired skin, follicles, and associated glands. They are often benign or low grade but can undergo malignant transformation with time.

Figure 1.18 shows a trichoepithelioma biopsy. Adnexal tumors, especially cystic adnexal tumors, are common, and are usually benign. They often grow around dilated follicles that fill with keratin. Evaluation of the epithelium lining the cyst wall is necessary for diagnosis of the tumor type and is critical for accurate prognosis. Manual extrusion of the cyst contents with biopsy of the keratin mass is unrewarding, as there will be no cyst wall present in the sample. Rupture of the cyst prior to removal can result in severe cellulitis with an influx of pleomorphic phagocytic cells (macrophages and multinucleate giant cells) that can almost appear to be a neoplastic population. FNA is appropriate prior to removal to rule out other more aggressive tumor types such as mast cell tumor. Removal of this tumor with at least 0.2 cm normal tissue at the margins is acceptable, and regrowth is not expected. Marginal excision ("shelling out") of the mass is not advisable because it may leave small amounts of tumor in the surgical bed to regrow or transform to a more aggressive form of this tumor.

Figure 1.19 shows a sebaceous adenoma biopsy. Proliferations of sebaceous glands are the fifth most common skin tumor of dogs and the eighth most common in cats.[8] They are characterized by proliferations of well-differentiated variably vacuolated sebaceous epithelial cells confined by a reserve cell lining of smaller basaloid epithelium, often around cystic and debris-laden ducts and follicles. Nomenclature based on the architectural arrangement of the cells includes sebaceous gland hyperplasia consisting of enlarging sebaceous gland epithelium rimmed by a single layer of basaloid epithelium extending from the follicle to ducts to the lobule, sebaceous adenoma consisting of proliferating sebaceous gland epithelium rimmed by a single layer of basaloid epithelium extending in a disorderly pattern from the duct and sebaceous epithelioma consisting of proliferating basaloid reserve cells around occasional foci of sebaceous gland epithelium that do not always clearly extend from a duct. These are listed from least aggressive to most aggressive in Table 1.4. Complete excision with conservative margins of at least 0.2 cm normal tissue is usually curative.

Figure 1.20 shows a sebaceous carcinoma biopsy. Sebaceous carcinoma is the malignant counterpart of benign sebaceous gland tumor and consists of poorly circumscribed proliferations of sebaceous gland and reserve basaloid cells that are not associated with ducts and invade into normal stroma. There is nuclear atypia with occasionally vesiculated chromatin, prominent nucleoli, and variably dense to vacuolated cytoplasm. A pre-surgical FNA finding of pleomorphic nuclei can be the hint that wide margins are necessary to achieve complete excision and allow enough marginal normal tissue to evaluate the adjacent lymphatics for invasion.

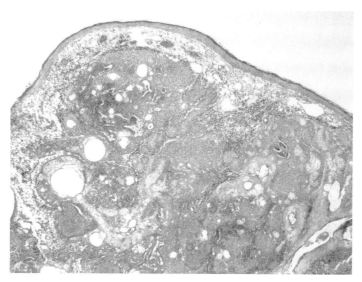

Figure 1.19 Sebaceous adenoma biopsy. 2.5x.

Table 1.4 Types of proliferations of sebaceous glands and the prognosis for each.

Category	Prognosis
Sebaceous hyperplasia	Benign
Sebaceous adenoma	Low grade
Sebaceous epithelioma	Low to mid grade
Sebaceous carcinoma	High grade, invasive

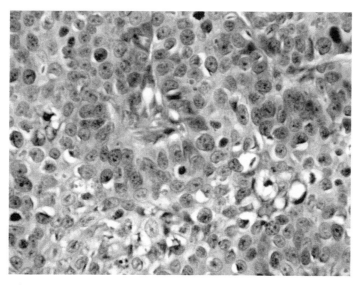

Figure 1.20 Sebaceous carcinoma biopsy. 40x.

Figure 1.21 shows a squamous cell carcinoma in situ biopsy. Carcinoma in situ (Bowen's disease) is seen mostly in cats and is a complex progression of pre-neoplastic to early neoplastic proliferations of squamous epithelial cells that are confined to the epidermis and do not cross the basement membrane into subepidermis. The epithelial cells can be pigmented with migration of melanophages and clumps of pigment into the underlying subepidermis. This lesion can be promoted by solar exposure (actinic keratosis) or papillomavirus infection, and can be multiple. If not completely excised it can progress to invasive carcinoma.

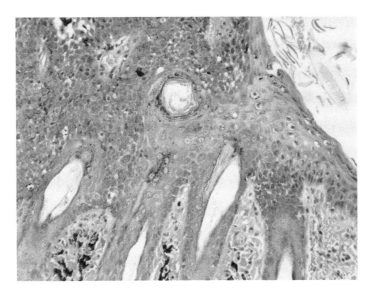

Figure 1.21 Carcinoma in situ biopsy. 10x.

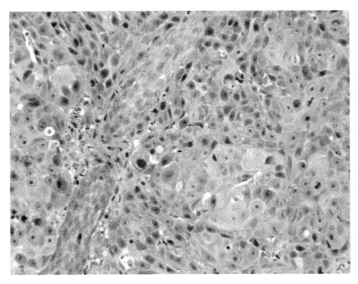

Figure 1.22 Squamous cell carcinoma biopsy. 20x.

Figure 1.22 shows a squamous cell carcinoma biopsy. Squamous cell carcinoma is a disorganized proliferation of variably keratinizing squamous epithelial cells that cross the basement membrane and invade into underlying stroma. They can be well differentiated, forming nodules of keratinizing cells (keratin pearls), or they can be anaplastic and form sheets of pleomorphic epithelioid cells. There is usually nuclear atypia with large nuclei, vesiculated chromatin, prominent, usually single, nucleoli and variable cytoplasmic keratinization, which is often asynchronous to nuclear maturation (dyskeratosis). This tumor type will readily invade stroma and local lymphatics, metastasizing to local lymph nodes and further. FNA can reveal these atypical morphologic features leading to a preliminary diagnosis of carcinoma. This can allow for referral to a specialist, or if referral is declined, can indicate a need for evaluation of local lymph nodes and thoracic radiographs, as well as wide surgical excision.

Epithelial tumors of the mucous membranes (mouth, conjunctiva, vagina, urinary bladder, intestine) can exhibit a rapid growth rate with early stromal invasion and may metastasize to lymph nodes readily. Notable exceptions are epulis and papilloma, which are usually benign, but can become locally invasive with time.

Figure 1.23 shows a canine epulis biopsy. This pink, firm gingival mass from a dog reveals anastomosing chains of epithelial cells extending from the epithelium into a proliferative fibrous stroma without visible breach of the interface

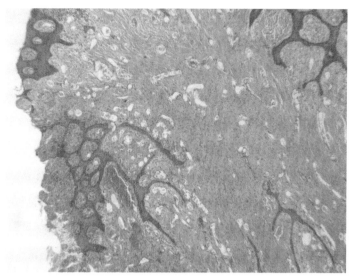

Figure 1.23 Canine epulis (peripheral odontogenic fibroma) biopsy. 2.5x.

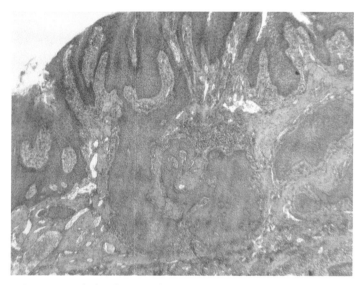

Figure 1.24 Canine ossifying acanthomatous epulis (ossifying acanthomatous ameloblastoma) biopsy. 2.5x.

basement membrane that would indicate stromal invasion. Complete excision of this low-grade biphasic lesion is often curative, but multiple foci may be present and additional masses may arise.

Figure 1.24 shows a canine ossifying acanthomatous epulis biopsy. This pink, firm gingival mass from a dog reveals a more proliferative epithelial component with occasional production of bone. It is a low-grade tumor and, although complete early excision may be curative, if not excised there is potential for invasion into and destruction of underlying bone. Radiographs prior to surgery would be helpful. Metastasis is not expected.

Figure 1.25 shows a canine oral papilloma biopsy. This oral mass was one of many excised from the mouth of a dog. The thickened, hyperkeratotic epithelium is thrown into folds over a fibrous stroma, and there is not stromal invasion. There may be viral inclusions and cytopathic changes in the epithelial cells. This lesion is often the result of papilloma-virus infection, it may be multiple, and additional lesions may arise. In an older dog with recurrent tumors, check for immunosuppression.

Figure 1.26 shows a canine conjunctival fibropapilloma biopsy. This tumor may be associated with trauma, and it tends to arise at the mucocutaneous junction of the eyelid. The cytopathic effects present in viral papillomas are not seen. Thickened and mildly dysplastic hyperkeratotic epithelium is thrown into folds over a loose fibrous stroma without stromal invasion. There is not significant hyperkeratosis. Viral genetic material is absent, and viral

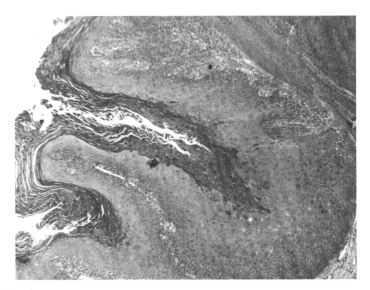

Figure 1.25 Canine oral papilloma biopsy. 2.5x.

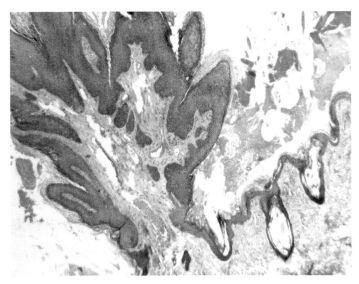

Figure 1.26 Canine conjunctival fibropapilloma biopsy. 2.5x.

antigens are not demonstrated. These lesions are often hyperpigmented and can be grossly similar to melanoma, thus the recommendation for removal when small.[9]

Figure 1.27 shows a canine urinary bladder transitional cell carcinoma biopsy. Biopsy evaluation of this bladder mass revealed a disorganized proliferation of pleomorphic epithelial cells with invasion into the underlying stroma. This tumor tends to metastasize to local lymph nodes and distant sites, but medical therapy can be palliative for a significant length of time with minimal complications in some dogs, and consultation with an oncologist for the most applicable and current therapy is suggested.

Figure 1.28 shows a squamous cell carcinoma of the nose biopsy. This disorganized proliferation of pleomorphic squamous epithelial cells exhibits nuclear atypia and stromal invasion. The central keratinization of some nests of cells is the identifying feature of this lesion.

Squamous epithelial tumors are often assessed by a combination of mitotic rate and invasion of stroma and lymphatics, and assigned a grade. Feline oral squamous cell carcinoma mitotic rates, however, appear not to be predictive of behavior, but stage, and especially the presence of bone invasion, is predictive.[10, 11] Radiographs, therefore, may have high prognostic significance in feline oral squamous cell carcinoma.

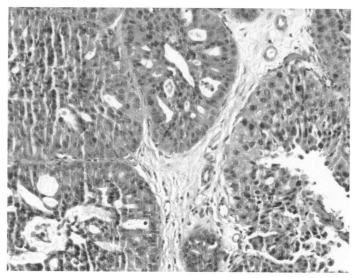

Figure 1.27 Canine urinary bladder transitional cell carcinoma biopsy. 10x.

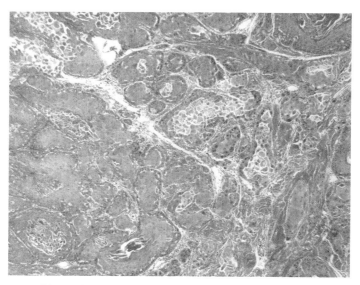

Figure 1.28 Squamous cell carcinoma of the nose biopsy. 40x.

Figure 1.29 shows a canine squamous cell carcinoma toe biopsy. This squamous cell carcinoma (arrow) in the toe of an adult dog has invaded into the third phalangeal bone causing disassociation of the joint cartilage (arrowhead). This suggests a high-grade tumor, and evaluation of local lymph nodes with thoracic radiographs would be part of the minimal database. Excision of the entire digit would remove this painful joint, which is unlikely to return to normal function, and may be necessary to achieve wide margins of normal tissue and provide assessment of bone and joint invasion.

Figure 1.30 shows a feline squamous cell carcinoma mouth biopsy. This squamous cell carcinoma from the mouth of an adult cat is forming a keratin pearl at the left margin and is clearly invasive into the stroma of the submucosa. The dense eosinophilic material at the lower right and upper left margins is bone and indicates that this tumor is invading the underlying bone. Mitotic figures are not seen in this field, but a high-grade tumor is suspected due to the bone invasion.

Tumors arising from epithelial cells of internal organs are often not discovered until a late stage. In one survey 76% of feline lung carcinomas had metastasized by the time of discovery.[12]

Figure 1.31 shows a lung bronchoalveolar carcinoma biopsy. Proliferation of atypical and disorganized bronchial lining epithelium can replace large areas of pulmonary parenchyma before clinical signs of respiratory distress are observed.

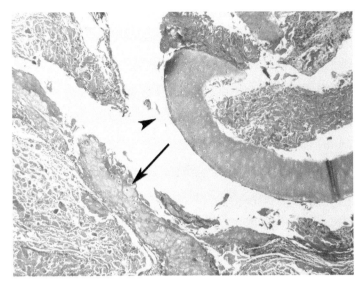

Figure 1.29 Canine squamous cell carcinoma toe biopsy. 2.5x.

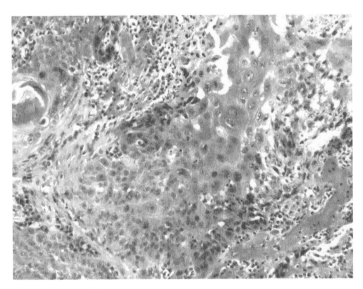

Figure 1.30 Feline squamous cell carcinoma mouth biopsy. 10x.

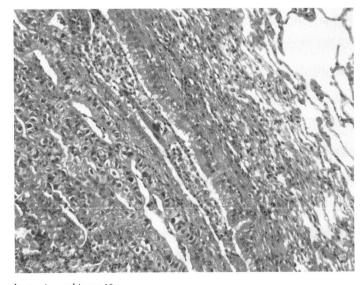

Figure 1.31 Lung bronchoalveolar carcinoma biopsy. 10x.

Figure 1.32 shows a biopsy of a pancreatic carcinoma metastatic to the liver. Ductular carcinoma in this adult female French Bulldog arose in the pancreas, metastasizing to adjacent organs including the liver as shown in this histologic section. There is both stromal (arrowheads) and lymphatic (arrows) invasion on this section. She presented with vague clinical symptoms, mostly anorexia, and a gastrointestinal foreign body was suspected. A pancreatic mass that had already spread to multiple other internal organs was found on exploratory laparotomy, and biopsy was performed postmortem.

Masses in internal organs may shed neoplastic cells into body cavity effusions. FNA of effusions is a rapid way to obtain a preliminary diagnosis. FNA of the mass can be performed prior to surgery if evaluation of an effusion is not diagnostic.

Figure 1.33 shows an intestinal adenocarcinoma FNA. An adult cat presented with abdominal effusion. FNA revealed clusters of epithelioid cells with marked anisokaryosis, prominent nucleoli, and basophilic cytoplasm that appear to contain fluid or mucin. When clusters of cells such as this are found free in the abdominal fluid, additional workup such as radiography or ultrasound is indicated to search for a mass that could be biopsied.

Figure 1.34 shows a biopsy of an intestinal mass in an adult cat that revealed invasion by glands from the lamina propria into the submucosa and muscular layers. These glands were lined by epithelial cells that were sometimes more than a single cell layer thick, with large pleomorphic nuclei exhibiting vesiculated chromatin with prominent nucleoli, and basophilic cytoplasm with large vacuoles. There was invasion into the local lymphatics by neoplastic rafts of cells with a similar morphologic appearance to the cells in Figure 1.33.

Mammary tumors can be composed of proliferating tubules and glands (simple), proliferating tubules, glands, and myoepithelial cells (complex), and proliferation of tubules, glands, myoepithelium and formation of cartilage and/or bone (mixed). Simple epithelial tumors are graded using type, nuclear pleomorphism, and mitotic rate, and this grade correlates with risk of invasion (see Table 1.3). Most canine mammary tumors are epithelial and myoepithelial (complex or mixed), however, and the grading system devised for simple mammary tumors is not applicable to complex or mixed tumors.[13] In dogs, ovariohysterectomy status and tumor grade, age, tumor stage, tumor subtype, and lymphatic metastasis were correlated with recurrence, metastasis, and survival time in one study and not related in another.[14, 15] Atypical ductal hyperplasia in dogs is associated with malignant neoplastic transformation, as is stromal invasion.[16] Fifty-three percent of feline mammary carcinomas had metastasized by time of discovery.[17] Mixed mammary tumors, the most common type of tumor found in dogs, tend to be less aggressive unless they are carcinosarcomas.[18] Mixed mammary tumors are not seen in cats.[19] It is difficult to evaluate stromal and lymphatic invasion if the tumor extends to all margins on the biopsy tissue submitted because one cannot look for invasion into normal adjacent stroma or lymphatics if neither is present. It is not advisable to "shell out" mammary tumors.

Figure 1.35 shows a biopsy from a young sexually intact female cat and reveals tubulolalveolar structures lined by a single layer of plump epithelium, which are then surrounded by laminar layers of myoepithelium. This is fibroepithelial hyperplasia, a benign response to hormonal stimulation and should regress upon removal of the hormonal stimulus.

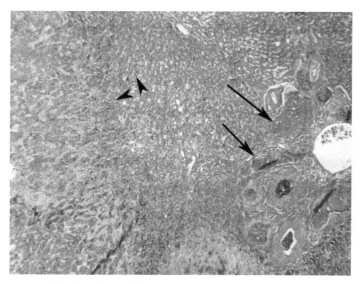

Figure 1.32 Pancreatic carcinoma metastatic to liver biopsy. 2.5x.

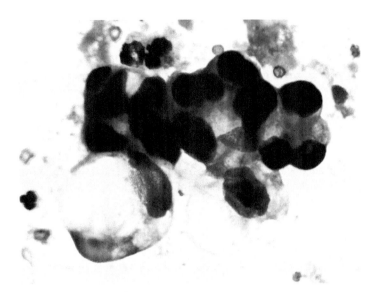

Figure 1.33 Intestinal adenocarcinoma in abdominal fluid FNA. 50x.

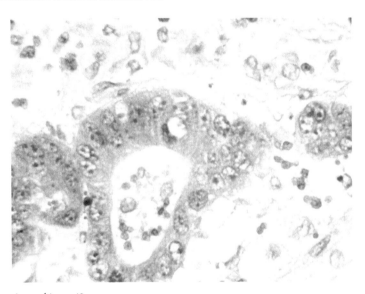

Figure 1.34 Intestinal adenocarcinoma biopsy. 40x.

Figure 1.36 shows a biopsy of a mammary adenoma on a middle-aged spayed female dog. It reveals a proliferation of tubuloepithelial cells in dilated ducts and glands. There is no stromal invasion seen, and adjacent lymphatics are not significantly dilated. Excision of this mass is indicated because benign tumors can eventually become invasive. Grossly recognizable normal tissue at the lateral margins and a tissue plane at the deep margin would be the minimal margin width warranted if pre-biopsy FNA does not reveal pleomorphic cells suggestive of a more aggressive tumor type. It is not advisable to "shell out" mammary tumors even if the FNA looks benign.

Figure 1.37 shows a biopsy of a mammary complex adenoma on a middle-aged spayed female dog and reveals a proliferation of tubuloepithelial cells in dilated ducts and glands with proliferation of associated myoepithelium. This is a complex tumor, and grading for simple tumors is not applicable. Complex tumors are usually low grade, but complete excision in a timely fashion is recommended because this tumor may undergo malignant transformation with time. Conservative margins of grossly normal tissue at the lateral margins and a tissue plane at the deep margin are indicated if there is not FNA evidence of cellular pleomorphism.

Figure 1.38 shows a biopsy of a mixed mammary tumor on a middle-aged sexually intact female mixed breed dog. It reveals a proliferation of tubuloepithelial cells in dilated ducts and glands with proliferation of associated myoepithelium, which is undergoing focal osseous and cartilaginous metaplasia. This tumor is low grade, but early excision is recommended because there is potential for malignant transformation with time. Conservative margins are indicated if there is not FNA evidence of cellular pleomorphism.

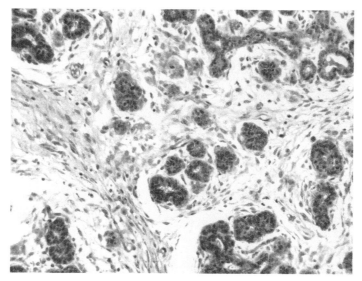

Figure 1.35 Feline mammary fibroepithelial hyperplasia biopsy. 10x.

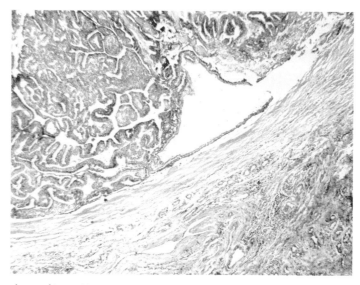

Figure 1.36 Canine mammary adenoma biopsy. 10x.

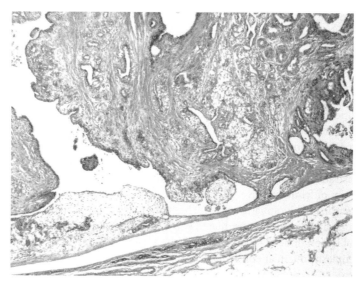

Figure 1.37 Canine mammary complex adenoma biopsy. 10x.

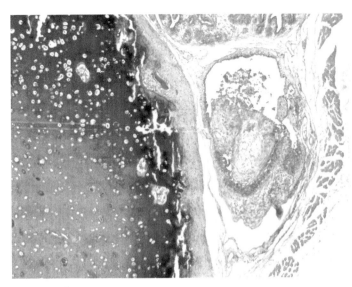

Figure 1.38 Canine mixed mammary tumor biopsy. 10x.

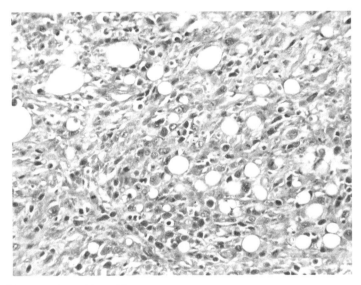

Figure 1.39 Canine invasive schirrous carcinoma biopsy. 10x.

Figure 1.39 shows a canine invasive schirrous carcinoma biopsy. This diffusely invasive mammary tumor in an adult female mixed breed dog exhibits nuclear pleomorphism, frequent mitotic figures, and loss of normal architecture. This type of tumor has a high potential for invasion into lymphatics and progression to distant sites. FNA of this type of tumor may yield pleomorphic cells that would confirm the need for thoracic radiographs prior to surgery. Complete excision with wide margins would allow a search for lymphatic invasion, and submission of local lymph nodes could be helpful for staging if there is lymphadenopathy.

Figure 1.40 shows a feline ductular carcinoma biopsy. This aggressive and high-grade tumor in an adult spayed female cat retained a somewhat duct-like appearance, but there is loss of normal lobular architecture and invasion into a fibrotic stroma. This type of tumor in the cat tends to invade lymphatics early. When taking a biopsy for initial diagnosis, wide margins are recommended so adjacent lymphatics can be searched for invasive tumor. Small biopsy samples may fail to demonstrate the invasive nature of the tumor.

Figure 1.41 shows a biopsy of feline invasive ductular carcinoma in the lymphatic structure. There are clusters of invasive ductular carcinoma in this lymphatic vessel. The wide margins of the tissue submitted, from the case in Figure 1.40, allowed demonstration of numerous dilated lymphatics containing invasive carcinoma.

Figure 1.42 shows a local lymph node that was also submitted with the tissue from Figure 1.40. There was invasion into the lymph node by neoplastic ductular epithelial cells.

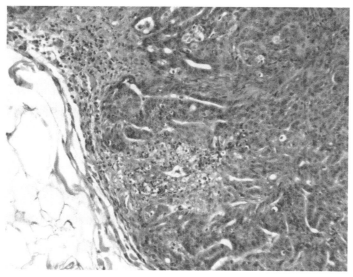

Figure 1.40 Feline ductular carcinoma biopsy. 10x.

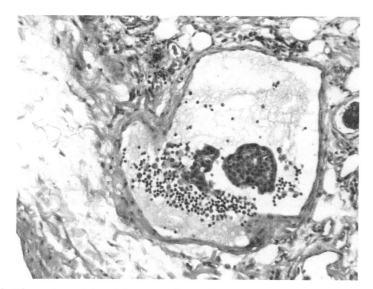

Figure 1.41 Feline invasive ductular carcinoma in lymphatic structure biopsy. 10x.

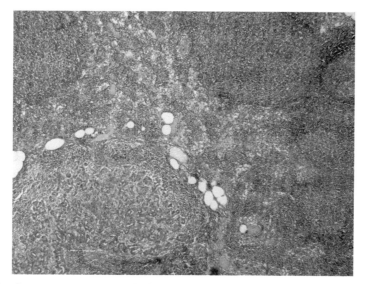

Figure 1.42 Feline invasive ductular carcinoma metastasis to local lymph node. 10x.

Mesenchymal tumors

Neoplasia of the stromal/spindle/mesenchymal cells of the body, also known as sarcoma when the proliferation is invasive, tends to be poorly circumscribed, as these cells are the framework of tissues and do not rest on a basement membrane. These tumors usually grow first by local extension then can metastasize to distant sites later in the course of the disease by hematogenous and lymphatic pathways. Mitotic rate and size of clean margins measured in millimeters (mm) or centimeters (cm) is predictive of behavior.[20] Complete removal of these tumors can be difficult to impossible depending on the location, and gross assessment of margins can be deceiving due to pseudoencapsulation and extension of fibrils along fascial planes. Tumor grade, mitotic rate and mitotic index, and size of clean margin are the most important prognostic indicators for spindle cell tumors.

Figure 1.43 shows a spindle cell tumor grade 1 biopsy. This biopsy from the skin of an adult dog reveals anastomosing bundles of cells that are typical of smooth muscle cells. Mitotic figures are 0–1/HPF with an MI of 1/10 HPF. There is no necrosis. This tumor would have a score of 1 + 1 + 1 = 3 and is a grade 1 tumor (Table 1.3).

Figure 1.44 shows a biopsy from the flank of an adult mixed breed dog is a disorganized proliferation of plump spindle cells of suspected nerve origin. There are 0–3 mitotic figures/HPF with an MI of 10/10 HPF. There are a few areas of necrosis, estimated at about 10% on the sample examined. This tumor would have a score of 2 + 2 + 2 = 6 and is a grade 2 tumor (Table 1.3).

Figure 1.45 shows a biopsy from the thigh of an adult beagle and is a disorganized proliferation of pleomorphic spindloid to epithelioid cells of indeterminate origin. There is moderate to marked anisokaryosis with prominent multiple nucleoli. There are 0–6 mitotic figures/HPF with an MI of 21/HPF. There is greater than 50% necrosis on the sections examined. This tumor would have a score of 3 + 3 + 3 = 9 and is a grade 3 tumor (Table 1.3).

Figure 1.46 shows a grade 2 spindle cell tumor. It was submitted with the history that excision appeared complete because there was normal tissue in the marginal tissue beyond the excised capsule. It is very important to note that spindle cell tumors do not form a capsule, and the bands that appear to be capsule are actually tumor.

Figure 1.47 shows a grade 2 spindle cell tumor that has less dense tissue at the margin, and this was assumed to be normal tissue based on the gross appearance. The black ink indicates the surgical margin. Tumor extends to the inked margin. Surgical removal of spindle cell tumors is fraught with peril. Referral for pre-surgical imaging and removal by a specialist should be offered because this tumor often extends widely microscopically. If referral is declined, any surgical removal should be performed with the knowledge that the tumor is likely to extend beyond the gross bulk of the mass.

Since many stromal or spindle cells have a similar appearance on routine histology, immunohistochemical stains may be necessary to identify the cell type (fibroblasts, pericytes, myopericytes, smooth muscle, myofibroblasts, Schwann cells, perineural cells) for optimum prognostic significance and treatment choices. Immunohistochemistry may be most useful when chemotherapy is a treatment option. This test is most satisfactory when performed on frozen tissue sections, but formalin fixed tissues are accepted and processed by many laboratories. Consultation with diagnostic

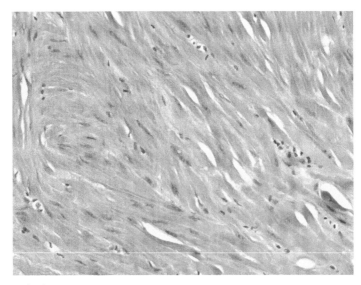

Figure 1.43 Spindle cell tumor grade 1 biopsy. 10x.

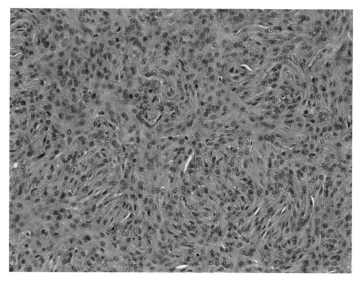

Figure 1.44 Spindle cell tumor grade 2 biopsy. 10x.

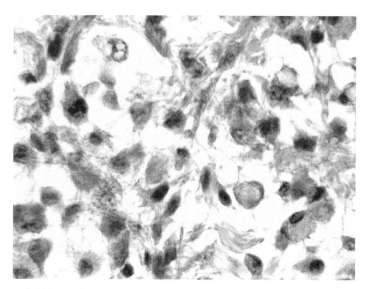

Figure 1.45 Spindle cell tumor grade 3 biopsy. 10x.

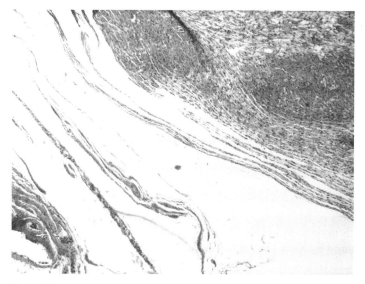

Figure 1.46 Spindle cell tumor biopsy. 2.5x.

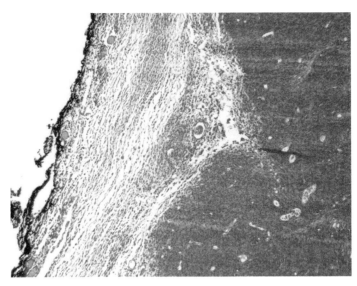

Figure 1.47 Spindle cell tumor biopsy. 2.5x.

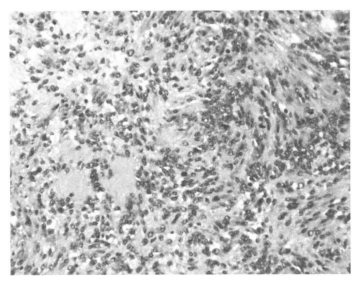

Figure 1.48 Spindle cell tumor biopsy. 10x.

lab personnel prior to submission is suggested for the most current information regarding test availability, submission requirements, and pricing. If chemotherapy will not be utilized and immunohistochemistry is not elected, then wide excision, with or without radiation therapy, is a standard therapy recommendation due to a similar biologic behavior for many soft tissue sarcomas.[21]

Figure 1.48 shows a grade 2 spindle cell tumor in a dog. The tumor exhibits a storiform pattern with occasional swirls and palisading nuclei when stained with routine hematoxalin and eosin (H&E) stain. This pattern is suggestive of neural tissue, and the tumor is presumed to be a peripheral nerve sheath tumor, but immunohistochemistry would be necessary for a more definitive diagnosis of the tumor cell type.

Figure 1.49 shows a grade 2 spindle cell tumor that is forming swirls and nests around vascular spaces, suggesting a peripheral vascular wall myocyte origin. Immunohistochemistry could be performed for more definitive identification of the tumor cell type.

Stromal/spindle cell tumors in cats can be aggressive no matter what the mitotic rate, with a recurrence rate of 14% for peripheral nerve sheath tumors diagnosed as benign and 31% for peripheral nerve sheath tumors diagnosed as malignant, based on one study.[22]

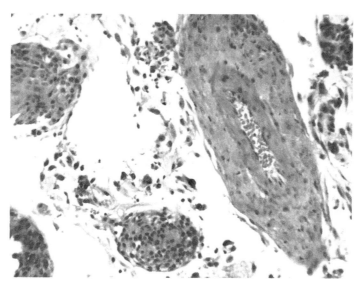

Figure 1.49 Spindle cell tumor biopsy. 10x.

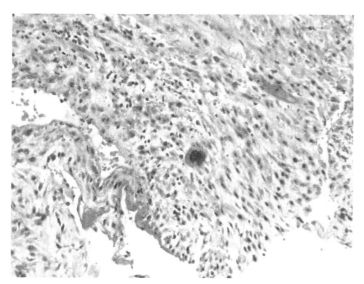

Figure 1.50 Feline soft tissue sarcoma. 10x.

Figure 1.50 shows a biopsy of a spindle cell tumor from an adult cat. It reveals many haphazardly arranged spindle cells and occasional large epithelioid cells with pleomorphic and lobulated nuclei, prominent nucleoli, and abundant cytoplasm. This cellular pleomorphism is the hallmark of feline soft tissue sarcomas and is a useful feature when evaluating a tumor using FNA, as the finding of even rare pleomorphic cells is an indication for immediate aggressive therapy.

Cutaneous hemangiosarcoma in dogs has a grading protocol that is based on a combination of mitotic rate and how deep the tumor extends, thereby estimating the potential for invasive behavior. Staging takes into account the presence of invasion beyond the local site. For example, stage I is confined to the dermis, stage II extends into subcutis and may exhibit regional lymph node involvement, and stage III invades structures such as muscle and involves distant metastasis.[23] Staging, while providing superior prognostic information, requires clinical information that cannot be determined from a single skin biopsy. Behavior in cats is unpredictable and ranges from locally invasive to aggressive and so attempts to grade may be misleading. Visceral hemangiosarcoma is quick to metastasize, and prognosis for long-term survival ranges from guarded with moderate to high probability of distant metastasis in non-ruptured tumors, to poor with a high probability of distant and local metastasis in ruptured tumors.[23] Benign hemangiomas can undergo malignant transformation to hemangiosarcoma with time, but complete early excision of hemangioma may be curative, so histopathological evaluation of all excised lesions suspected of being vascular in origin is very important in order to confirm clean margins.

Figure 1.51 is a cutaneous hemangiosarcoma in an adult dog and consists of a somewhat circumscribed mass composed of vascular channels lined by pleomorphic endothelium. There were 0–2 mitotic figures/HPF. It was confined to the dermis and was considered to be low grade due to the relatively low mitotic rate and minimal local invasion.

Figure 1.52 shows a hepatic hemangiosarcoma, diagnosed at necropsy in an adult male Weimaraner. This was likely a metastatic lesion, as there was hemangiosarcoma in the spleen, and hemo-abdomen was observed upon opening the abdominal cavity. Preliminary diagnosis was made by identifying abdominal fluid on ultrasound and confirming abundant free blood by FNA.

The most common bone tumor is canine osteosarcoma. Behavior (time until metastasis and survival time) appears to be correlated to the site of occurrence. Bone tumors of the head and jaw tend to metastasize less readily than other sites. Osteosarcoma of the scapula has a significantly greater hazard for death than appendicular sites. Every 100% increase in alkaline phosphatase (ALP) increases the hazard of death by 1.7, and tumor grade at this site is not predictive according to one report.[24] Osteochondromatosis, a benign lesion, was reported to undergo malignant transformation

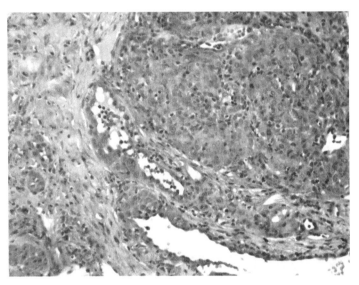

Figure 1.51 Canine cutaneous hemangiosarcoma. 10x.

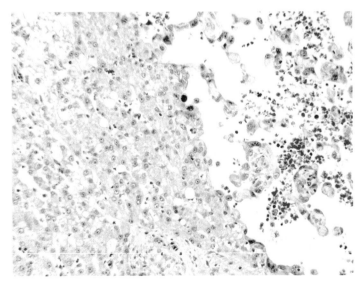

Figure 1.52 Canine hepatic hemangiosarcoma. 10x.

to chondrosarcoma over a course of 20 months in one reported case.[25] Spontaneous regression of osteosarcoma has also been reported.[26] Due to the many variables associated with predicting the behavior of this tumor type, consultation with an oncologist would be prudent.

Figure 1.53 An adult mixed breed dog presented with a firm mass on the left dorsal skull that on biopsy consisted of well-differentiated cartilage and bone with lacunae containing osteocytes and chondrocytes with small nuclei. This is typical of a benign or low-grade bone tumor such as osteochondroma. Metastasis is not expected, and complete excision may be curative.

Figure 1.54 shows a biopsy of an adult German Shepherd Dog presented with a mass near the orbit. Biopsy reveals a haphazard proliferation of bone, cartilage, and occasional sheets of pleomorphic spindloid to epithelioid cells diagnosed as osteosarcoma. This tumor is moderately well differentiated, producing tumor bone, and at this site is unlikely to produce early metastasis. Euthanasia was elected due to the extreme deformation of the skull and ocular involvement.

Figure 1.55 shows a biopsy of an adult Mastiff presented with left front leg lameness. Radiographs revealed a lytic lesion of the left humerus, and biopsy revealed a proliferation of pleomorphic epithelioid cells with rare multinucleated cells. Some cells appear to be nestled within scant eosinophilic material suggestive of osteoid, supporting a

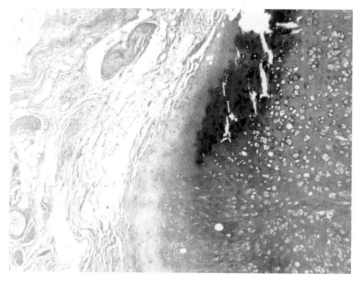

Figure 1.53 Osteochondroma biopsy. 2.5x.

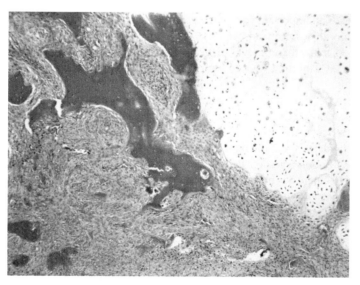

Figure 1.54 Osteosarcoma biopsy. 2.5x.

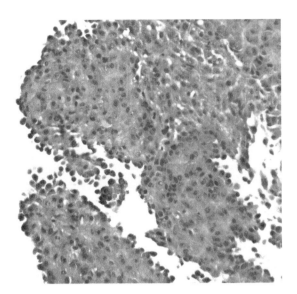

Figure 1.55 Osteosarcoma biopsy. 10x.

diagnosis of osteosarcoma. Definitive diagnosis of this tumor with evaluation of mitotic rate can be difficult if small samples from core biopsies are submitted, as this tumor can form in close association with necrotic bone, reactive bone, and periosteal hyperplasia, creating a heterogeneous pattern that can lead to sampling error. It can be a challenge to obtain a sample of adequate size and diagnostic quality without creating a site of instability.

Round cell tumors

Canine mast cell tumors (MCT) have historically been graded with a three-part system historically referred to as the Patnaik system.[27] Grade 1 (low-grade tumors) have 0 mitotic figures/HPF, are well differentiated, and are confined to the subepidermis and superficial dermis. Grade 2 (mid-grade tumors) have 0–2 mitotic figures/HPF, rare binucleate cells, and are dermal to subcutaneous. Grade 3 (high-grade tumors) have three or more mitotic figures/HPF, are pleomorphic, and extend to subcutaneous or deeper tissues.

A more recent system developed at Michigan State University by Kiupel et al. (which will be referred to as the two-tier scale), uses a two-part grading protocol in which a high-grade tumor is diagnosed if there are >7 mitosis/10 HPF, 3 multinucleated cells in 10 HPF, or 3 bizarre nuclei in 10 HPF and a low-grade tumor is diagnosed if these conditions are not met.[28] Mitotic index is an important part of the grading process of both systems, with one study indicating an MI < 5/10 HPF had a 70-month survival and MI > 5/10 HPF had 2-month survival.[29] In a study comparing the two systems over a 5-year period, in the three-level (Patnaik) grading system there was 0% mortality due to tumors labeled grade 1 (low grade, 1 of 3) 23% mortality due to tumors labeled grade 2 (mid grade, 2 of 2), and 100% mortality in tumors labeled grade 3 (high grade, 3 of 3). In the two-tier grading system there was 6% mortality due to tumors labeled low grade (1 of 2) and 71% mortality due to tumors labeled high grade (2 of 2), and the newer two-tier system was deemed to be more clinically predictive on a statistical basis.[30]

Figure 1.56 shows a canine cutaneous mast cell tumor grade 1 Patnaik scale. This cutaneous canine mast cell tumor is confined to the superficial dermis, mitotic figures are rare, and the mast cells appear well differentiated with small, monomorphic nuclei. This tumor is a grade 1 Patnaik scale tumor and a low-grade two-tier scale tumor (Table 1.2).

Figure 1.57 shows a canine cutaneous mast cell tumor grade 2 Patnaik scale. There are variably granulated mast cells with small but slightly pleomorphic nuclei, 0–1 mitotic figures/HPF with an MI of 2/10 HPF, and the tumor extends to the deep dermis. This tumor would be a grade 2 Patnaik scale and a low-grade two-tier scale (Table 1.2).

Figure 1.58 shows a canine cutaneous mast cell tumor grade 2 Patnaik scale. This grade 2 (Patnaik), low-grade (two- tier) cutaneous mast cell tumor has small, variably granulated mast cells with small nuclei with mild anisokaryosis, and is confined to the dermis. There are areas of collagen necrosis with dense infiltrates of eosinophils. Identification of mitotic figures is difficult in these areas, and they should be avoided because the irregular appearance of eosinophil nuclei could cause a spurious elevation in the mitotic count.

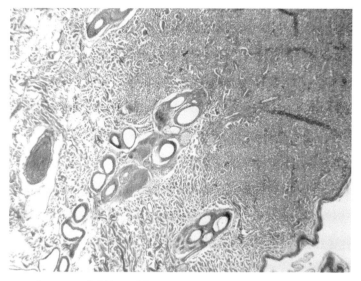

Figure 1.56 Canine cutaneous mast cell tumor grade 1 biopsy. 2.5x.

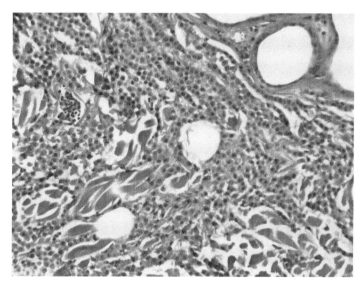

Figure 1.57 Canine cutaneous mast cell tumor grade 2 biopsy. 10x.

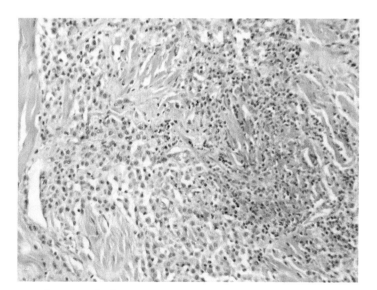

Figure 1.58 Canine cutaneous mast cell tumor grade 2 biopsy. 10x.

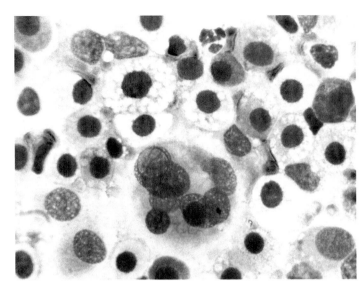

Figure 1.59 Canine mast cell tumor FNA. 50x.

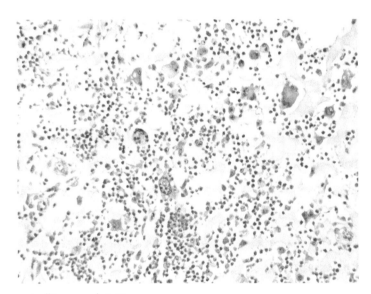

Figure 1.60 Canine cutaneous mast cell tumor grade 3. 40x.

Figure 1.59 shows the aspirate of a mass from a six-year-old spayed female Mastiff dog that revealed pleomorphic mast cells with moderate to marked anisokaryosis and frequent cells with multiple nucleoli, prominent nucleoli in some cells, and variable cytoplasmic granulation. Note that most of the cells are larger than the neutrophil in the top middle right and lymphocyte at the top middle left. There is not a grading system applicable to aspirates, but this tumor is likely to be high grade on biopsy due to the extreme cellular pleomorphism.

Figure 1.60 shows a canine cutaneous mast cell tumor grade 3 Patnaik scale. This biopsy of the aspirated mass in Figure 1.59 reveals a proliferation of moderately pleomorphic mast cells with identifiable cytoplasmic granules, and numerous large epithelioid cells without distinct cytoplasmic granules and with marked anisokaryosis and multiple nucleoli in an edematous background. This tumor extended into subcutaneous tissue and to all margins. There were low numbers of mitotic figures, but the extensive invasion of deep tissues and extreme cellular pleomorphism suggested a diagnosis of grade 3 Patnaik scale, high-grade two-tier scale, mast cell tumor (Table 1.2). Giemsa stain was recommended for confirmation that the pleomorphic cells were mast cells.

Figure 1.61 shows a canine cutaneous mast cell tumor grade 3 Patnaik, Giemsa stain. Giemsa stain of the biopsy in Figure 1.60 reveals metachromatic granules in the giant epithelioid cells, revealing them to be anaplastic mast cells. This tumor is confirmed as a grade 3 Patnaik scale and high-grade two-tier scale mast cell tumor.

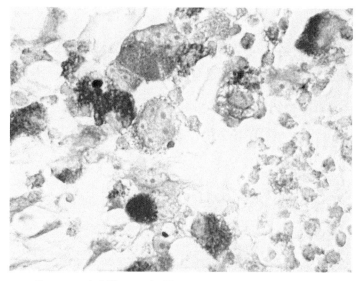

Figure 1.61 Canine cutaneous mast cell tumor grade 3 Giemsa stain. 50x.

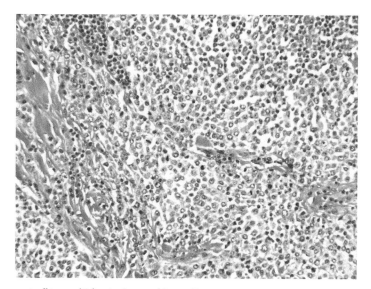

Figure 1.62 Canine cutaneous mast cell tumor high mitotic count biopsy. 10x.

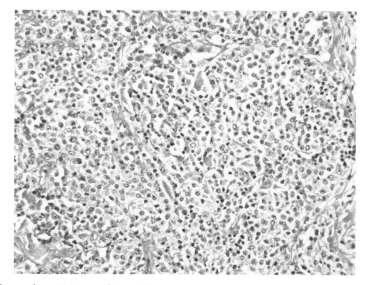

Figure 1.63 Canine mast cell tumor low mitotic count biopsy. 10x.

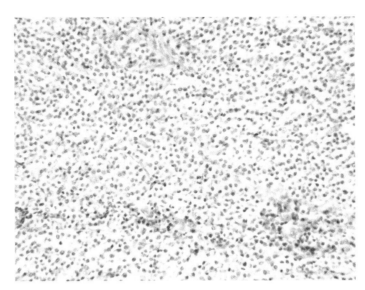

Figure 1.64 Feline cutaneous mast cell tumor biopsy. 10x.

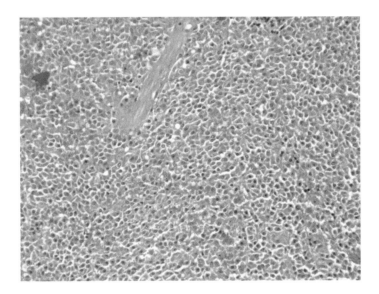

Figure 1.65 Feline splenic mast cell tumor biopsy. 10x.

In the study that comparatively assessed tumors with both the two-part (low, high) and three-part (1, 2, 3) systems, all grade 1 MCTs were diagnosed as low grade, all grade 3 MCTs were diagnosed as high grade, and 82% of grade 2 MCTs were diagnosed as low grade with 18% of grade 2 MCTs diagnosed as high grade. It should be noted that regarding the clinical relevance of this study, the mortality rate for two-tier low-grade MCT was 6%, and the mortality rate for two-tier high-grade MCT was 71%, while the mortality rate for Patnaik grade 1 was 0%, grade 2 was 23%, and grade 3 was 100%. Grading of MCT does not predict behavior with 100% accuracy, but both systems were significantly associated with prognosis, and there was greater concordance among pathologists when the two-tier system was used.[30]

Figure 1.62 shows a cutaneous mast cell tumor that was graded as a grade 3 Patnaik, high-grade two-tier, due to the many mitotic figures in a certain area of the tumor. There appears to be nine or more mitotic figures in this field.

Figure 1.63 shows the same cutaneous mast cell tumor seen in Figure 1.62. The mitotic rate is low in this field, and most of the irregular nuclei are eosinophils. This demonstrates one source of variability in grading, because some tumors have areas of significant variation in the density of mitotic figures.

Canine mast cell tumors with tyrosine kinase receptor (KIT) dysregulation may behave in a more aggressive fashion.[31] Feline mast cell tumors do not reveal a prognostic association with KIT expression, and there is no recognized grading system, but higher mitotic rates are suggestive of more aggressive behavior.[32]

Figure 1.64 is a biopsy from an adult cat with a skin mass that revealed sheets of mast cells with rare mitotic figures. There is not a grading system applicable to feline mast cell tumors at this time. Complete excision of this type of lesion is often curative.

Figure 1.65 shows the splenic biopsy from an adult cat with a diffusely enlarged spleen. This is an indication for immediate diagnostic workup. The complete blood count (CBC) can be searched for circulating mast cells, and evaluation of abdominal fluid for mast cells is also an appropriate procedure prior to surgery. Mast cells are not normally seen in these fluids, and the finding of more than rare mast cells in the CBC or abdominal fluid is supportive of splenic mast cell tumor when there is splenomegaly. FNA of the spleen can be performed if these tests are not diagnostic. Also check for skin masses and palpate lymph nodes, and perform thoracic radiographs. Splenectomy is the treatment of choice with reported remission times of 12–19 months. Degranulation of splenic mast cell tumor can lead to fatal hypotension so gentle handling is important.[33]

Malignant lymphoma (lymphosarcoma) grading is still a work in progress, but there are generalizations that seem to be useful across the many types of lymphomas. Lymph node lymphoma and extranodal lymphoma have site-specific biological behavior. Canine hepatosplenic T-cell lymphoma and hepatic T-cell lymphoma are poorly responsive to therapy at this time, and they usually behave in an aggressive biological fashion.[34, 35] Low-grade T-cell lymphoma at a number of sites including skin and liver can be indolent, and quality of life can be maintained without aggressive therapy for long periods of time.[36]

Grading of nodal lymphomas is predominantly based on mitotic rate with 0–5/HPF graded low, 6–10/HPF graded intermediate, and >10/HPF graded high.[1, 37] In one retrospective study, dogs with low-grade T-cell lymphoma had a median survival rate of 622 days, dogs with high grade T-cell lymphoma had a median survival rate of 162 days, and dogs with B-cell centroblastic, the most common type, had a median survival rate of 127–221 days, across multiple treatment protocols.[1] Identification of T- and B-cell types is important for prognosis and therapeutic plan, and can be performed on biopsy samples by immunohistochemistry and on FNA samples using flow cytometry or polymerase chain reaction (PCR) of antigen receptor site rearrangements (PARR). Reactive hyperplasia may progress to low-grade or high-grade lymphosarcoma.[38] In cases where definitive diagnosis of neoplasia is difficult due to a morphologically heterogeneous lymphocyte population as determined by FNA or biopsy, antigen receptor site rearrangement PCR (PARR) can identify clonal populations that would support a diagnosis of neoplasia.[39] In cats, lymphoma prognosis is significantly affected by both retroviral infection and site of the neoplasm.[40]

Figure 1.66 shows a reactive lymph node biopsy. Enlarged lymph nodes can be a result of follicular hyperplasia due to antigenic stimulation. There should be multiple well-circumscribed cortical nodules composed of germinal centers of B-cell origin lined by a wall of more dense small lymphocytes of mostly T-cell origin. The medullary sinusoids should be well defined and contain plasma cells and small lymphocytes. FNA will usually reveal a mixed population of small and large lymphocytes. Progression from reactive hyperplasia to neoplasia has been reported.

Figure 1.67 shows a biopsy of a lymph node with lymphoma that reveals loss of the normal follicular architecture with replacement of the follicles and sinusoids by sheets of monomorphic lymphocytes. This low-grade lymphoma exhibits few mitotic figures.

Figure 1.68 shows a biopsy of a high-grade lymphoma that reveals loss of architecture similar to Figure 1.67, but there will be many mitotic figures.

Figure 1.69 shows a cutaneous lymphoma. Cutaneous lymphoma can be seen in many skin locations from haired skin to mucosal surfaces. In epitheliotrophic cutaneous T-cell lymphoma, the most diagnostically helpful feature of this tumor is finding invasion into the epidermal layer by neoplastic round cells. Biopsy samples must have some intact epidermis to identify this trait.

Figure 1.70 shows a splenic malignant lymphoma biopsy. Histologic evaluation of a diffusely enlarged spleen revealed sheets of T-cell lymphocytes. This tumor type is often aggressive and generally responds poorly to therapy, although low-grade, slow-growing types have been reported.[34, 35]

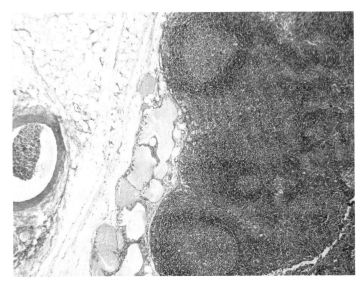

Figure 1.66 Reactive lymph node biopsy. 2.5x.

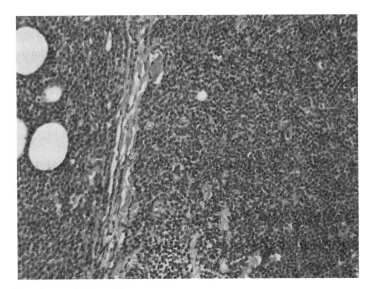

Figure 1.67 Lymph node lymphoma, low-grade biopsy. 10x.

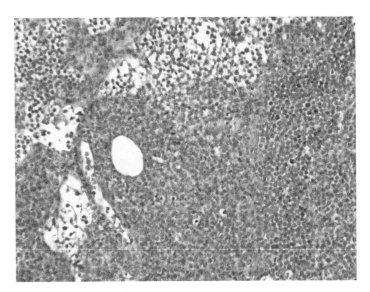

Figure 1.68 Lymph node lymphoma, high-grade biopsy. 10x.

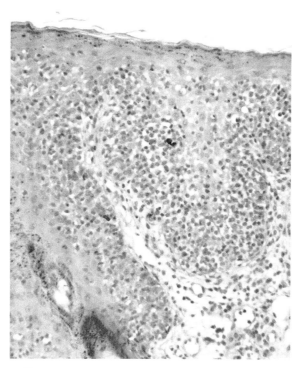

Figure 1.69 Cutaneous lymphoma biopsy. 10x.

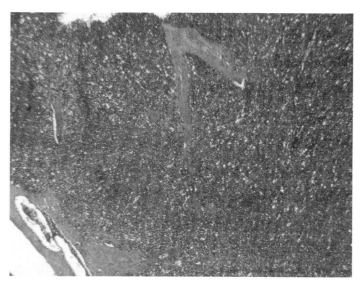

Figure 1.70 Splenic malignant lymphoma biopsy. 10x.

Histiocytic tumors are especially complicated.[41] Histiocytoma is a round cell tumor seen most often in young dogs. It may spontaneously regress, but cases have been reported of multifocal lesions progressing to histiocytosis, on rare occasions even invading local lymph nodes prior to regressing. Histiocytic sarcoma is the malignant form of this tumor. Benign cutaneous histiocytoma is not reported in the cat, but progressive histiocytosis and histiocytic sarcoma are known to occur. Histiocytic neoplasia tends to be staged rather than graded.

Canine histiocytic sarcoma arising in internal organs reportedly had a metastatic rate of 66% and a median survival time of 14.4 to 43.6 days whereas tumors of the limbs had a metastatic rate of 28% and a median survival time of 125.6 to 164.4 days.[42] Feline progressive histiocytosis and Langerhan's cell histiocytosis are progressive and debilitating. The feline proliferations can be reactive or neoplastic, but both exhibit relentless progression.[43]

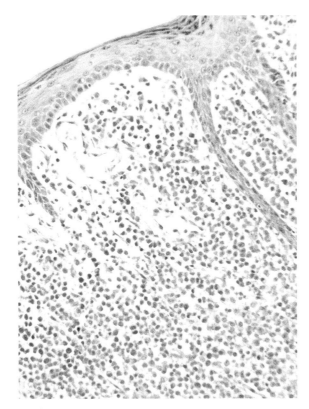

Figure 1.71 Canine cutaneous histiocytoma biopsy. 10x.

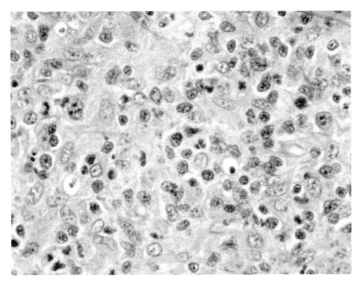

Figure 1.72 Canine cutaneous histiocytosis biopsy. 40x.

Figure 1.71 shows a canine cutaneous histiocytoma biopsy. Canine cutaneous histiocytoma often presents as an ulcerated dome-shaped mass composed of sheets of histiocytes with fairly monomorphic round to reniform nuclei, scattered mitotic figures, bland chromatin, and moderate pale cytoplasm. They are often arranged in loose arrays extending up to the epidermis, sometimes with epidermal invasion. At the margins there are often foci of small lymphocytes and plasma cells.

Figure 1.72 shows a biopsy of canine cutaneous histiocytosis. A clinical history of multiple, sometimes waxing and waning, epithelioid cell infiltrates with moderately pleomorphic nuclei and abundant coarse cytoplasm is typical of histiocytosis. Immunohistochemistry would be necessary for definitive diagnosis of the tumor type.

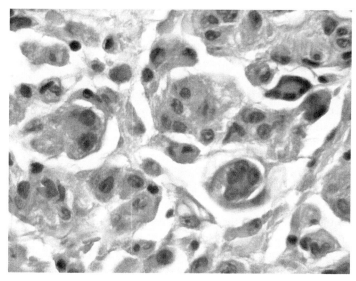

Figure 1.73 Histiocytic sarcoma biopsy. 40x.

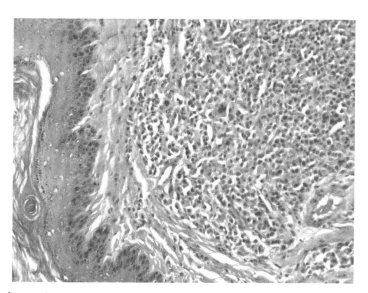

Figure 1.74 Plasma cell tumor biopsy. 10x.

Figure 1.73 shows a histiocytic sarcoma biopsy. This adult male Schnauzer was presented for a subcutaneous mass on the thorax. Biopsy revealed areas of spindle cells with a storiform pattern interspersed with areas of epithelioid and multinucleate cells. There were 0–3 mitotic figures/HPF with 12 mitotic figures/10 HPF. The mass extended to surgical margins. The epithelioid and multinucleate cells are suggestive of histiocytic lineage, and a presumptive diagnosis of histiocytic sarcoma was made. Confirmation of the cell type with immunohistochemistry was advised. Thoracic and abdominal radiographic and ultrasound evaluation, complete laboratory evaluation, and examination of local lymph nodes is advised due to the tendency of this tumor type to spread widely. Additional imaging modalities could be helpful if thoracic radiographs are negative. Consultation with a specialist for the most current therapeutic protocol is suggested.

Plasma cell tumor is a common round cell tumor in the skin of dogs, and is sometimes seen in cats. It is usually benign in spite of a pleomorphic appearance to the cells, but malignant forms can occur. Prognosis is best correlated to two factors: factor one being if there are tumor cells infiltrating bone and internal organs with associated hypercalcemia, and factor 2 being if there is production of serum or urine myeloma proteins with subsequent organ damage due to hyperviscosity.[44] The presence of either factor lowers the prognosis.

Figure 1.74 shows a plasma cell tumor biopsy. This dome-shaped hairless skin mass on an adult female Bulldog was biopsied and revealed many round cells with eccentric nuclei and numerous binucleate and trinucleate cells with occasional cells exhibiting large lobular nuclei with dense chromatin. This nuclear pleomorphism is a diagnostic feature of benign plasma cell tumor.

Melanoma

In the canine species, melanoma prognosis is heavily influenced by location and mitotic rate.[45] Melanomas located on a mucosal surface tend to be aggressive and metastasize readily, but benign forms can occur. Melanomas on haired skin tend to be more indolent and metastasize later in the course of the disease, but highly aggressive tumors can occur. Skin tumors with a mitotic index of less than 3/10 HPF tend to be less aggressive and are often benign, and oral tumors with a MI of less than 4/10 HPF tend to be lower grade, which means that complete excision with greater than 0.5-cm margins and no evidence of lymphatic or distant spread could be curative.[46] Since this tumor can undergo malignant transformation with time, large slow growing tumors can develop areas of high mitotic activity as they age, and the area of highest mitotic rate should be chosen for evaluation. Ultimately prognosis involves site, size of tumor, grade, and width of clean margins after removal.

In the feline species behavior is unpredictable, and the completeness of the excision is likely to have the most effect on survival.

Figure 1.75 shows a well-differentiated tumor that exhibits deeply pigmented tumor cells in the subepidermal region. No mitotic figures are seen in the less well-pigmented areas. There is junctional activity with at least 0.2 cm normal tissue at the margins, which suggests complete excision of this low-grade tumor although ideally at least 0.5 cm of normal tissue at the lateral margins and 1 fascial plane deep is the preferred minimal margin.[45, 46]

Figure 1.76 shows a melanoma biopsy with junctional activity (arrows). Junctional activity (nested proliferations of the neoplastic melanocytes) is a distinguishing feature of the melanoma. It can only be evaluated if there is intact skin present so submission of completely ulcerated lesions can delay definitive diagnosis in poorly differentiated tumors.

Figure 1.77 shows a biopsy of cutaneous melanoma that is well differentiated. This variably pigmented proliferation of melanocytes demonstrates 0–1 mitotic figures/HPF with an MI of 2/10 HPF. There is junctional activity at the interface in some areas. This tumor is considered to be a well-differentiated tumor.

Figure 1.78 shows a biopsy of cutaneous melanoma that is poorly differentiated. This poorly pigmented proliferation of pleomorphic epithelioid to spindloid cells exhibits marked anisokaryosis and multilobular nuclei. Overall MI was 19, although there are only scattered mitotic figures in this field. These cells are not clearly of melanocyte origin, and the presence of junctional activity at the epidermal interface is necessary for definitive diagnosis without resorting to immunohistochemistry. Samples taken from ulcerated areas may not have any epithelium, resulting in an inability to look for junctional activity. This tumor type has a high probability for metastasis and/or regrowth so an accurate diagnosis is critical.

Figure 1.79 is an FNA of a pleomorphic, poorly differentiated melanoma that reveals a spindle cell with minimal melanin and an epithelioid cell with moderate melanin. This pleomorphism in a population is a hallmark of melanoma.

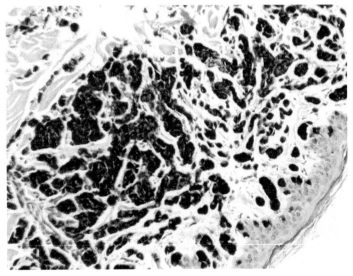

Figure 1.75 Well differentiated dermal melanoma of canine skin biopsy. 10x.

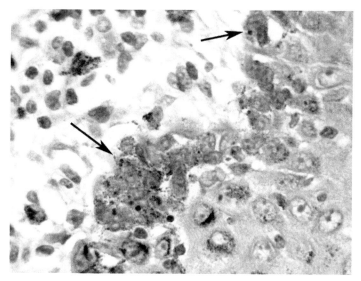

Figure 1.76 Melanoma biopsy showing junctional activity. 40x.

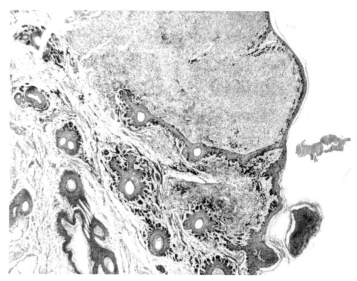

Figure 1.77 Cutaneous melanoma well-differentiated biopsy. 2.5x.

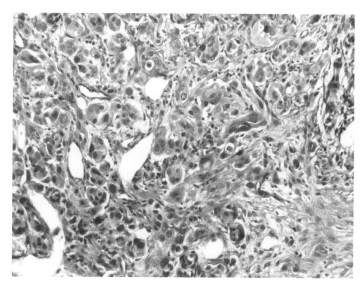

Figure 1.78 Cutaneous melanoma poorly differentiated biopsy. 10x.

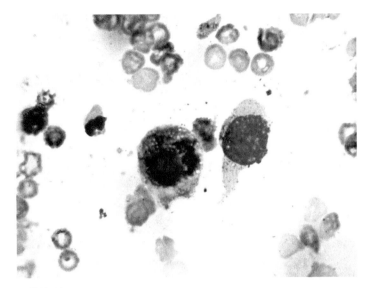

Figure 1.79 Cutaneous melanoma FNA. 50x.

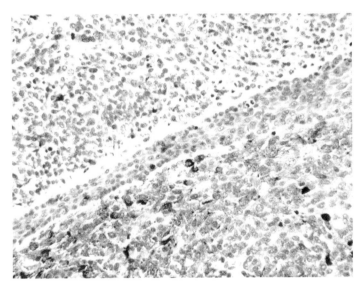

Figure 1.80 Cutaneous melanoma, poorly differentiated biopsy. 10x.

Figure 1.80 shows a biopsy of poorly differentiated melanoma that reveals a heterogeneous population of poorly pigmented spindloid melanocytes adjacent to a population of more deeply pigmented melanocytes in the same tumor, demonstrating the cellular pleomorphism seen in the aspirate in Figure 1.79. Biopsy at different sites can yield a very different appearing tumor.

Conclusion

In conclusion, some tumors are significantly influenced by location, others by mitotic rate, and others by multiple factors such as reproductive hormone receptors, hypoxia, and tyrosine kinase receptor expression (KIT).[47, 48] Benign tumors can grow large without becoming aggressive, can become malignant and metastasize, or sometimes can spontaneously disappear. Malignant tumors can contain populations of benign or reactive cells, confusing the diagnosis, and reactive populations can sometimes look malignant histologically. For the owner with limited funding, or the owner who declines referral, treatment by the general practitioner with antibiotics such as doxycycline for infectious diseases that cause immune dysfunction and chronic reactive lymphoid proliferations, cyclooxygenase (COX) inhibitors for epithelial tumors, tyrosine kinase inhibitors for mast cell tumors (MCT) and gastrointestinal stromal tumors (GIST) that exhibit receptor alterations, judicious use of immunosuppressives for lymphoproliferative diseases, and excision with clean margins, may result in extension of lifespan with a good quality of life. Consultation with a specialist regarding current therapy recommendations may yield the most satisfactory results because this field is rapidly advancing and the published literature can experience some delay. For the owner with high expectations, testing beyond basic histopathology (immunohistochemistry, antigen receptor site rearrangement PCR, c-KIT analysis for the specified (KIT) tyrosine kinase receptor mutation, silver staining of nucleolar organizer regions (Ag-NOR), and other developing procedures) is likely necessary to provide adequate information for proper therapy.

A few key points regarding some common tumors can be useful to the general practitioner.

Epithelial tumors tend to be more aggressive when simple (one cell type such as a purely glandular tumor) as opposed to compound (for example, epithelial and myoepithelial populations as in a mixed mammary tumor). The location can be predictive (squamous cell carcinoma may be invasive earlier at mucosal sites than at haired skin sites). And invasion by epithelial tumors into adjacent stroma and lymphatics, and especially bone, is generally a bad prognostic indicator.

Histiocytic tumors in any location have a poor prognosis in cats, but in dogs the location is strongly correlated with behavior (cutaneous histiocytoma versus splenic histiocytic sarcoma).

Lymphoid neoplasia prognosis can be correlated to cell type. B-cell tumors tend to be rapidly expansive, in both dogs and cats, while T-cell tumors can be aggressive or indolent (slow growing) with the mitotic rate predictive of behavior in dogs.

Mast cell tumor behavior correlates to grade, which is significantly influenced by mitotic rate and nuclear pleomorphism in dogs. In cats there is not a currently accepted grading protocol predictive of behavior, but site (skin versus internal organs) and mitotic rate can affect behavioral characteristics.

Melanoma morbidity and mortality are most affected by complete excision, and the mitotic rate and degree of nuclear pleomorphism are valuable prognostic indicators.

Sarcomas in dogs also can be best mitigated by early wide excision, and mitotic rate and cellular pleomorphism are strongly correlated to behavior. In cats certain sarcomas, sometimes associated with tissue injury due to various causes, are highly aggressive and location is predictive in that the ability to completely amputate the affected area with wide margins can increase survival time.

References

1. Valli VE, Kass PH, Myint MS, Scott F. Canine lymphomas: Association of Classification Type, Disease Stage, Tumor Subtype, Mitotic Rate, and Treatment with Survival. Vet Path 2013; 50:738–748.
2. Kamstock DA, Ehrhart EJ, Getzy DM. Recommended Guidelines for Submission, Trimming, Margin Evaluation, and Reporting of Tumor Biopsy Specimens in Veterinary Surgical Pathology. Vet Path 2011; 48:19–31.
3. Clifford C, Skorupski K, Moore P. Histiocytic diseases. In Small Animal Clinical Oncology, 5th ed. Withrow and MacEwen. 2013. Elsevier. St. Louis. 706–715.
4. Smedley RC, Spangler WL, Esplin DG, Kitchell BE, Bergman PJ, Ho H-Y, Bergen IL, Kiupel M. Prognostic Markers for Canine Melanocytic Neoplasms: A Comparative Review of the Literature and Goals for Future Investigation. Vet Path 2011; 48:54–72.
5. Sorenmo KU, Rasotto R, Zappulli V, Goldschmidt MH. Development, Anatomy, Histology, Lymphatic Drainage, Clinical Features, and Cell Differentiation Markers of Canine Mammary Gland Neoplasms. Vet Path 2011; 48:85–97.
6. Vail DM, Pinkerton ME, Young KM. Hematopoietic Tumors. In Small Animal Clinical Oncology, 5th ed. Withrow and MacEwen. 2013. Elsevier. St. Louis. 608–627.
7. Sorenmo KU, Worley DR, Goldschmidt MH. Tumors of the Mammary Gland. In Small Animal Clinical Oncology, 5th ed. Withrow and MacEwen. 2013. Elsevier. St. Louis. 538–556.
8. Hauck ML. Tumors of the Skin and Subcutaneous Tissues. In Small Animal Clinical Oncology, 5th ed. Withrow and MacEwen. 2013. Elsevier. St. Louis. 306.
9. Beckwith-Cohen B, Teixeira LBC, Ramos-Vara JA, Dubielzig RR. Squamous Papilloma of the Conjunctiva in Dogs: A Condition Not Associated with Papillomavirus Infection. Vet Path 2015; 52:676–680.
10. Belluco S, et al. Digital Squamous Cell Carcinoma in Dogs, Epidemiological, Histological, and Immunohistochemical Study. Vet Path 2013; 50:1078–88.
11. Theon AP, Madewell BR, Shearn VI, et al. Prognostic factors associated with radiotherapy of squamous cell carcinoma of the nasal plane in cats. JAVMA 1995; 206:991–996.
12. Hahn KA, McEntee MF. Primary lung tumors in cats: 86 cases (1979–1994). JAVMA 1997; 211:1257–1260.
13. Rasotto R, Zappulli V, Castagnaro M, Goldschmidt MH. A Retrospective Study of Those Histopathologic Parameters Predictive of Invasion of the Lymphatic System by Canine Mammary Carcinomas. Vet Path 2012; 49:330–340.

14. Pena L, De Andres PJ, Clemente M, et al. Prognostic Value of Histological Grading in Noninflammatory Canine Mammary Carcinomas in a Prospective Study With Two-Year Follow-Up: Relationship With Clinical and Histological Characteristics. Vet Path 2013; 50:94–105.

15. Pena L, Gama MH, Goldschmidt MH. Canine Mammary Tumors: A Review and Consensus of Standard Guidelines on Epithelial and Myoepithelial Phenotype Markers, HER2, and Hormone Receptor Assessment Using Immunohistochemistry. Vet Path 2014; 51:127–145.

16. Ferreira E, Gobbi H, Saraiva BS, Cassali GD. Histological and Immunohistochemical Identification of Atypical Ductal Mammary Hyperplasia as a Preneoplastic Marker in Dogs. Vet Path 2012; 49:322–329.

17. Penafiel-Verdu C, Buendia AJ, Navarro JA, et al. Reduced Expression of E-cadherin and B-catenin and High Expression of Basal Cytokeratins in Feline Mammary Carcinomas with Regional Metastasis. Vet Path 2012; 49:979–987.

18. Goldschmidt M, Pana L, Rasotto R, Zappulli V. Classification and Grading of Canine Mammary Tumors. Vet Path 2011; 48:117–131.

19. Zappulli V, Caliari D, Rasotto R, et al. Proposed Classification of the Feline "Complex" Mammary Tumors as Ductal and Intraductal Papillary Mammary Tumors. Vet Path 2013; 50:1070–77.

20. Dennis MM, McSporran KD, Bacon NJ, et al. Prognostic Factors for Cutaneous and Subcutaneous Soft Tissue Sarcomas in Dogs. Vet Path 2011; 48:73–84.

21. Liptak JM, Forrest LJ. Soft tissue sarcomas. In Small Animal Clinical Oncology, 5th ed. Withrow and MacEwen. 2013. Elsevier. St. Louis. 356–369.

22. Schulman FY, Johnson TO, Facemire PR, Fanburg-Smith JC. Feline Peripheral Nerve Sheath Tumors: Histologic, Immunohistochemical, and Clinicopathological Correlation (59 Tumors in 53 Cats). Vet Path 2009; 46:1166–1180.

23. Thamm D. Hemangiosarcoma. In Small Animal Clinical Oncology, 5th ed. Withrow and MacEwen. 2013. Elsevier. St. Louis. 679–688.

24. Kruse MA, Holmes ES, Balko JA, et al. Evaluation of Clinical and Histopathologic Prognostic Factors for Survival in Canine Osteosarcoma of the Extracranial Flat and Irregular Bones. Vet Path 2013; 50:704–708.

25. Aeffner F, Weeren R, Morrison S, et al. Synovial Osteochondromatosis with Malignant Transformation to Chondrosarcoma in a Dog. Vet Path 2012; 49:1036–1039.

26. Mehl ML, Withrow SJ, Seguin B, et al. Spontaneous remission of osteosarcoma in four dogs. JAVMA 2001; 219:614–617.

27. Patnaik AK, Ehler WJ, MacEwen EG. Canine Cutaneous Mast Cell Tumor: Morphologic Grading and Survival Time in 83 Dogs. Vet Path 1984; 21:469–474.

28. Kuipel M, Webster JD, Bailey KL, et al. Proposal of a 2-Tier Histologic Grading System for Canine Cutaneous Mast Cell Tumors to More Accurately Predict Biological Behavior. Vet Path 2011; 48:147–155.

29. Romansik EM, Reilly CM, Kass PH, et al. Mitotic Index Is Predictive for Survival for Canine Cutaneous Mast Cell Tumors. Vet Path 2007; 44:335–341.

30. Vascellari M, Giantin M, Capello K, et al. Expression of Ki67, BCL-2, and COX-2 in Canine Cutaneous Mast Cell Tumors: Association With Grading and Prognosis. Vet Path 2013; 50:110–121.

31. Zemke D, Yamini B, Yuzbasiyan-Gurkan V. Mutations in the Juxtamembrane Domain of c-KIT Are Associated with Higher Grade Mast Cell Tumors in Dogs. Vet Path 2002; 39:529–535.

32. Sabattini S, Guadagni Frizzon M, Gentilini F, et al. Prognostic Significance of Kit Receptor Tyrosine Kinase Dysregulations in Feline Cutaneous Mast Tumors. Vet Path 2013; 50:797–805.

33. London CA, Thamm DH. Mast Cell Tumors. In Small Animal Clinical Oncology, 5th ed. Withrow and MacEwen. 2013. Elsevier. St. Louis. 346–349.

34. Fry MM, Vernau W, Pesavento PA, et al. Hepatosplenic lymphoma in a dog. Vet Path. 2003. 40:556–562.

35. Keller SM, Vernau W, Hodges J, et al. Hepatosplenic and Hepatocytotropic T-Cell Lymphoma: Two Distinct Types of T-Cell Lymphoma in Dogs. Vet Path. 2012; 50:281–290.

36. Vail DM, Pinkerton ME, Young KE. Hematopoietic tumors. In Small Animal Clinical Oncology, 5th ed. Withrow and MacEwen. 2013. Elsevier. St. Louis. 608–638.

37. Valli VE, Myint MS, Barthel A, et al. Classification of canine malignant lymphomas according to the World Health Organization criteria. Vet Path. 2011; 48:198–211.

38. Valli VE, Vernau W, de Lorimier P, et al. Canine indolent nodular lymphoma. Vet Path. 2006; 43:241–256.

39. Burnett RC, Vernau W, Modiano JF, et al. Diagnosis of Canine Lymphoid Neoplasia Using Clonal Rearrangements of Antigen Receptor Genes. Vet Path. 2003; 40:32–41.

40. Vail DM, Pinkerton ME, Young, KE. Hematopoietic tumors. In Small Animal Clinical Oncology, 5th ed. Withrow and MacEwen. 2013. Elsevier. St. Louis. 638–653.

41. Moore PF. A Review of Histiocytic Diseases of Dogs and Cats. Vet Path 2014; 51:167–184.

42. Constantino-Casas F, Mayhew D, Hoather TM, Dobson JM. The Clinical Presentation and Histopathologic-Immunohisto-chemical Classification of Histiocytic Sarcomas in the Flat Coated Retriever. Vet Path 2011; 48:764–771.

43. Busch MDM, Reilly CM, Luff JA, Moore PF. Feline Pulmonary Langerhans Cell Histiocytosis with Multiorgan Involvement. Vet Path 2008; 45:816–824.

44. Vail DM. Myeloma-Related Disorders. In Small Animal Clinical Oncology, 5th ed. Withrow and MacEwen. 2013. Elsevier. St. Louis. 365–378.

45. Bergman PJ, Kent MS, Farese JP. Melanoma. In Small Animal Clinical Oncology, 5th ed. Withrow and MacEwen. 2013. Elsevier. St. Louis. 321–334.

46. Campagne C, Jule S, Alleaume C, et al. Canine Melanoma Diagnosis: RACK1 as a Potential Biological Marker. Vet Path 2013; 50:1083–1090.

47. Abbondati E, Del-Pozo J, Hoather TM, et al. An Immunohistochemical Study of the Expression of the Hypoxia Markers Glut-1 and Ca-IX in Canine Sarcomas. Vet Path 2013; 50:1063–69.

48. Maes RK, Langohr IM, Wise AG, et al. Beyond H&E: Integration of Nucleic Acid-Based Analysis Into Diagnostic Pathology. Vet Path 2014; 51:238–256.

PART II

Case Studies

2 Selected Lesions of the Head and Neck

Bone tumors of the head

Masses arising from the bone of the calvarium and periorbital area are often not recognized until there is significant distortion of the skull, as there tends to be no discharge, bleeding, or pain evidenced. Fine needle aspiration (FNA) can give a preliminary description of the proliferating cell types, but biopsy is required for definitive diagnosis because the elements of reactive bone can be cytologically indistinguishable from well-differentiated neoplastic bone.

Figure 2.1 shows a clinical presentation of a hard mass over the frontal sinus area of an adult female spayed Labrador mix. There is significant distortion of the skull (arrow). FNA of this type of lesion can reveal bone elements that will be regular in appearance if this is a low-grade bone lesion or may reveal atypical bone elements if this is a malignant bone tumor. Radiographs are suggested to look for bone proliferative or lytic regions that would be a good location for aspiration or biopsy. FNA can identify cells typical of those responsible for bone production, but without clearly atypical cells biopsy is needed to evaluate the architecture.

Osteoma

Figure 2.2 shows a canine osteoma. Aspiration of a periorbital mass in an adult spayed female mixed breed dog revealed a background of blood with a large osteoclast (arrow) and many epithelioid osteoblasts (arrowheads) with regular nuclei. These are cells typically seen in proliferating bone and do not indicate if the bone is reactive versus neoplastic. Biopsy is suggested for definitive diagnosis.

Figure 2.3 shows a canine multilobular tumor of the bone. A 10-year-old intact female Golden Retriever was presented with a hard mass on top of the head at the left occipital protuberance, extending caudally and laterally toward the back of the skull. It had grown over a period of 5–7 weeks. It was debulked and submitted. The specimen was a $3.5 \times 2.5 \times 2.5$ cm portion of a bony somewhat granular mass. The specimen was decalcified whole. The outer surface was multilobular, smooth, and tan/brown. A representative section from the center was processed for histology. The mass had a multilobular or multinodular architecture. It is comprised by contiguous bony lobules bordered by septa of spindle cells. The nodules are comprised of bone and cartilage. The lobules vary in size, and cartilaginous differentiation predominates in many of the lobules in the representative section. Mitotic index (MI) = 1/10 high-power field (HPF). Groups of multinucleated cells are scattered among the lobules and nodules. The mass extends into the deep margin of the section. Multilobular tumors of bone can become locally aggressive, they often recur even if they appear to have been completely resected, and some of them eventually undergo malignant transformation to osteosarcoma. The osteosarcomas can metastasize via blood vessels and lymphatics. Skull is the most common site for this tumor type in canines. These tumors have a very characteristic radiographic appearance.

Osteosarcoma

Figure 2.4 shows a canine osteosarcoma. Aspiration of a variably lytic to proliferative lesion of the zygomatic bone in an adult spayed female mixed breed dog reveals blood and scattered epithelioid cells compatible with osteoblasts (arrowhead) that exhibits moderate to marked anisokaryosis. There is a focus of cells nested within eosinophilic matrix that is suggestive of osteoid. The variation in nuclear size is the distinguishing feature that suggests that this population is neoplastic.

Atlas for the Diagnosis of Tumors in the Dog and Cat, First Edition. Anita R. Kiehl and Maron Brown Calderwood Mays.
© 2016 John Wiley & Sons, Inc. Published 2016 by John Wiley & Sons, Inc.

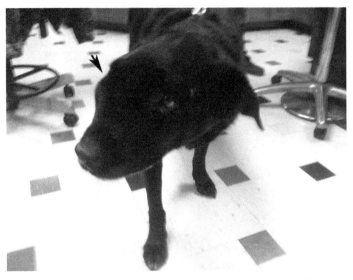

Figure 2.1 Clinical photograph of a hard mass over the frontal sinus area of an adult female spayed Labrador mix.

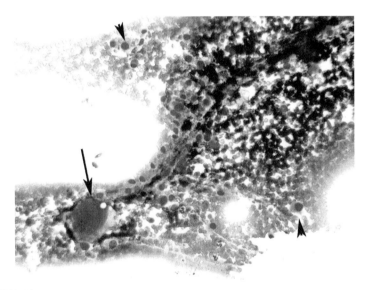

Figure 2.2 Canine osteoma FNA. 10x.

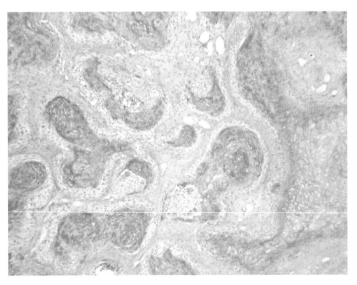

Figure 2.3 Canine multilobular tumor of bone biopsy. 4x.

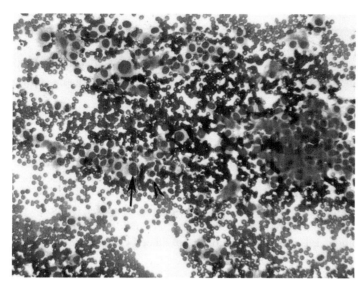

Figure 2.4 Canine osteosarcoma FNA. 10x.

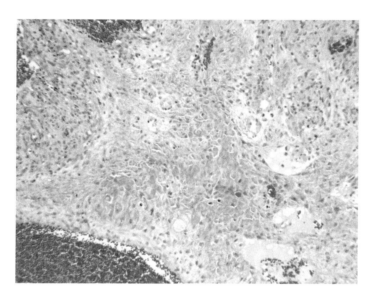

Figure 2.5 Feline telangiectatic osteosarcoma. 10x.

Figure 2.5 shows feline telangiectatic osteosarcoma. A rapidly enlarging 2-cm subcutaneous mass developed over the left eye of a 16-year-old Domestic Shorthair cat in a period of 2 months. No osseous destruction was noted on radiographs. A $2.0 \times 1.0 \times 1.7$ cm portion of a multilobular brown/tan mass was submitted. The mass is a pleomorphic mesenchymal neoplasm. It is comprised by medium to large polygonal cells with considerable variation in cell and nuclear size, at least one prominent nucleolus, and a moderate amount of eosinophilic cytoplasm with indistinct cell borders. These cells multifocally deposit osteoid, and there are fragments of well-differentiated bone embedded in the mass. Other bony trabeculae are poorly differentiated and immature. Similar cells also line anastomosing blood-filled spaces. Ischemic necrosis is focally extensive. Hematoidin deposits and siderocytes in some areas indicate past hemorrhage. In solid areas mitoses are seen at a rate of up to 3/HPF, and abnormal mitotic figures are present. Rare mitoses are seen in the cells lining blood-filled spaces, and these cells occasionally have double nuclei. Margins could not be accurately assessed. This pleomorphic sarcoma is most consistent with telangiectatic osteosarcoma. Osteosarcomas are locally aggressive, they can recur even if completely resected, and they metastasize readily to the lungs and then to other organs in many species. They occasionally spread to regional lymph nodes, as well. Osteosarcomas are slower to metastasize in felines than in canines, but the prognosis should still be considered poor because of the location and the poor circumscription of the primary mass.

Mass lesions of the ear canal

Polypoid masses can be found in the ear canal of dogs and cats. The most common types of masses are benign polyps (dog and cat) and benign and malignant ceruminous gland tumors (cat). FNA followed by biopsy is an appropriate clinical approach, as the finding of pleomorphic cells on FNA would suggest the need for wide surgical margins and evaluation of draining lymph nodes.

Aural polyp

Figure 2.6 shows a feline ear canal polyp. Aspiration of a polyp in the ear canal of a 3-year-old male Persian cat yielded a mixed population of slender spindle cells, epithelial cells with typical small nuclei from the mucosal surface, active macrophages from around dilated ceruminous glands, and variably pigmented surface debris. The cellularity should be low, and nuclei should be small and monomorphic.

Figure 2.7 shows a feline ear canal polyp biopsy. A 12-year-old female spayed Calico cat presented with a nodular ear canal mass that was removed and submitted for histologic evaluation. Variably ulcerated mucosa covers a firm proliferation of slender spindle cells around low numbers of dilated ceruminous glands (arrows) with periglandular infiltrates of small lymphocytes, plasma cells, and macrophages. There appears to be normal tissue at the margins. Complete excision is often curative.

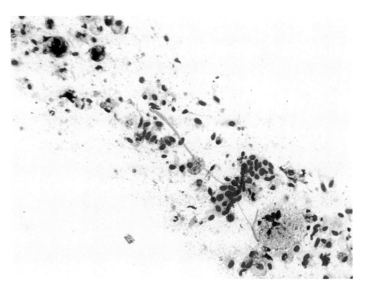

Figure 2.6 Feline ear canal polyp FNA. 10x.

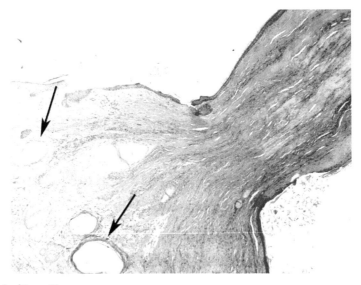

Figure 2.7 Feline ear canal polyp biopsy. 10x.

Ceruminous adenoma

Figure 2.8 shows canine ceruminous adenoma. Aspirate of an ear canal mass in an adult female Boston Terrier dog reveals clusters of regular appearing cuboidal epithelium with small monomorphic nuclei and moderate pale to lightly basophilic cytoplasm that can form chains and acini in a background of scant blood and free nuclei. The regular appearance of the epithelial cells and small monomorphic nuclear size suggests a benign behavior, but this tumor type can become aggressive with time so early complete excision with biopsy is recommended.

Figure 2.9 shows canine ceruminous adenoma. An 11-year-old neutered male Weimaraner developed a bleeding friable mass in the right ear. Friable small brown/tan microlobular specimens were submitted and processed for histology. There was thick well-differentiated stratified squamous epithelium on the outer surface, indicating external ear canal origin. The mass is an epithelial neoplasm comprised by small to medium polygonal and cuboidal cells that form many branching tubules lined by one and sometimes two layers of crowded cells. Potential mitoses are infrequent. Margins could not be assessed. Canine ceruminous gland neoplasms are usually benign in behavior, at least for extended periods of time, and the cells comprising this one appear bland and benign. Complete resection is the treatment of choice. However, the tumors can recur if not completely resected.

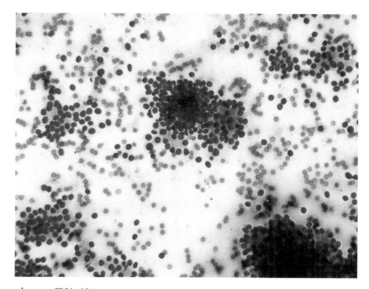

Figure 2.8 Canine ceruminous adenoma FNA. 10x.

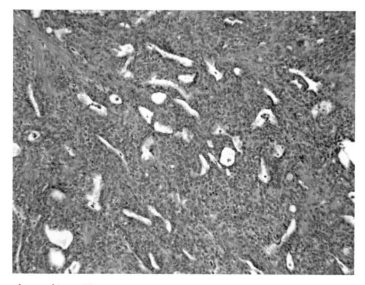

Figure 2.9 Canine ceruminous adenoma biopsy. 10x.

Ceruminous carcinoma

Figure 2.10 shows feline ceruminous carcinoma. Aspiration of a persistent mass in the ear canal of a aged spayed female Domestic Shorthair cat reveals many epithelioid cells with moderate to marked anisokaryosis, prominent nucleoli, and basophilic cytoplasm in a background of neutrophils and macrophages. This degree of nuclear pleomorphism is a hallmark of aggressive neoplasia, and timely removal of the mass with biopsy and evaluation for clean margins is recommended.

Figure 2.11 shows feline ceruminous carcinoma. A 5-year-old spayed female Domestic Shorthair cat was presented with an aural mass previously biopsied elsewhere and found to be a ceruminous gland adenocarcinoma. A total ear canal ablation was performed, and the left ear canal was submitted. A representative section through the mass was processed for histology. The mass was ulcerated. It was poorly circumscribed, and the stroma was infiltrated by neutrophils, lymphocytes, and plasma cells. The mass is comprised of branching sometimes dilated tubules lined by enlarged and somewhat pleomorphic multilayered polygonal, cuboidal, and columnar epithelial cells of apocrine type. Some of these tubules are filled with neutrophils. There are smaller infiltrative more solid aggregates of similar neoplastic cells. Identifiable margins on the sections were clean. Ceruminous gland tumors are malignant in behavior over 50% of the time in cats (unlike in dogs.) They can recur even if completely resected, and they are also capable of metastasis via lymphatics at a later date.

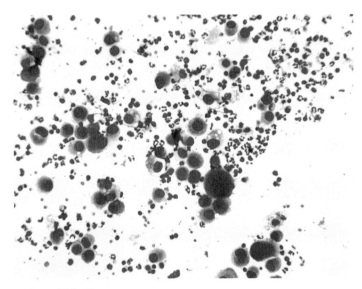

Figure 2.10 Feline ceruminous carcinoma FNA. 10x.

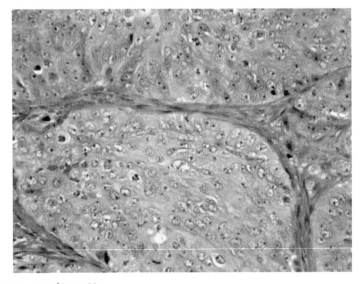

Figure 2.11 Feline ceruminous carcinoma biopsy. 20x.

Mass lesions of the external ear pinna

Circumscribed masses can be seen on the canine ear pinna. FNA prior to surgery is prudent because there is little room on the ear pinna for wide deep margins, and diagnosis of a benign or low-grade lesion may spare surgical resection of the ear.

Histiocytoma

Figure 2.12 shows a canine histiocytoma. This dense round cell population from a button-like mass on the ear pinna of a 9-month-old Bulldog is composed of cells slightly larger than an accompanying lymphocyte. These round cells exhibit fine chromatin, round to occasionally reniform nuclei, and pale to lightly basophilic cytoplasm. If this mass persists or becomes multiple, biopsy is recommended for confirmation.

Figure 2.13 shows canine histiocytoma of the ear pinna. A raised cutaneous mass had been noted on the outer surface of the left pinna of a 12-year-old spayed female Labrador Retriever for more than 8 months when she was presented.

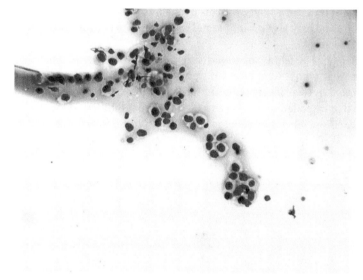

Figure 2.12 Canine histiocytoma FNA. 10x.

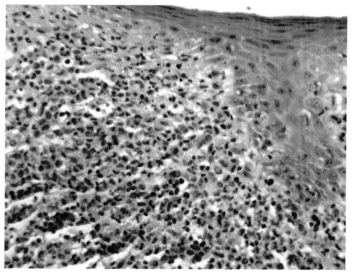

Figure 2.13 Canine histiocytoma, ear pinna. 20x.

The owner allowed biopsies only, and two biopsies were submitted. The mass is composed of sheets of histiocytic cells. The cells at the dermal-epidermal junction are more loosely arranged. The mitotic rate is moderate. The cells are agranular and unpigmented. Margins could not be accurately assessed. This round cell tumor is histologically consistent with histiocytoma. Skin of the ear pinna is a common site. These tumors are usually benign and solitary, often occurring in young dogs. However, the tumors can develop anywhere on the body at any age, and they can recur if not completely resected.

Squamous cell carcinoma

Figure 2.14 shows a clinical presentation of a white cat with bilateral surgically removed ear tips due to squamous cell carcinoma. Poorly circumscribed to diffuse lesions on the ears of cats should be superficially scraped and the cell type evaluated prior to biopsy. The most common lesion seen at this site, especially in a white cat, is squamous cell carcinoma, but melanoma, spindle cell tumor, and mast cell tumor can also be seen.

Figure 2.15 shows a feline squamous cell carcinoma. A 2-year-old white male neutered cat was presented with crusty ear tips. Cytologic exam of a scraping revealed many squamous epithelial cells with moderate to marked anisokaryosis, prominent nucleoli, and abundant clear to lightly basophilic cytoplasm. The large nuclei and nucleoli demonstrate asynchronous maturation with the clear cytoplasm. This is a hallmark of squamous cell carcinoma. This lesion may be exacerbated by solar exposure and may prove multiple and recurrent with continued solar exposure. Bacteria may grow in the ulcerated surface (arrowheads).

Figure 2.16 shows a biopsy of a feline squamous cell carcinoma. An adult male neutered cat had ulcerated bleeding lesions on the ear tips, which were biopsied, revealing a disorganized proliferation of squamous epithelial cells with moderate to marked nuclear pleomorphism, nuclear and cytoplasmic dysmaturation, 0–5 mitotic figures/HPF, and stromal invasion that extended to the margins of the tissue submitted. Wide resection of both ear pinnas was recommended. Complete excision, if prior to nodal metastasis, can result in extended survival times.

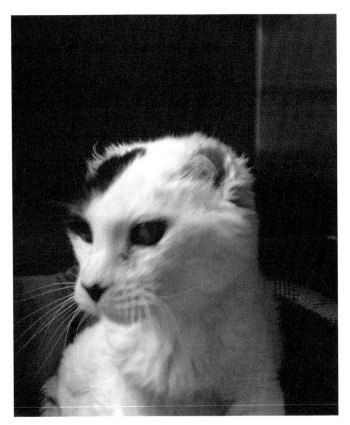

Figure 2.14 Clinical photograph of a white cat with bilateral surgically removed ear tips due to squamous cell carcinoma.

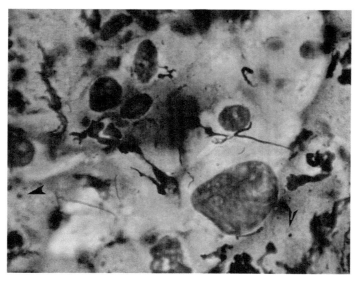

Figure 2.15 Feline squamous cell carcinoma FNA. 50x.

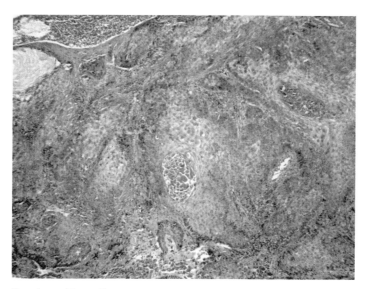

Figure 2.16 Feline squamous cell carcinoma biopsy. 10x.

Mass lesions of the conjunctiva and nictitans

Lesions on the conjunctiva and external structures of the eye are often seen early in the course of the disease. Cytologic exam, usually of slides made from the scraped surface, can be useful to determine if the process is inflammatory and requires medical therapy, or if the mass is a neoplastic proliferation and should be removed with histologic evaluation.

Papilloma

Figure 2.17 shows canine conjunctival papilloma. Cytologic exam of a scraping of a conjunctival papillary lesion on the left lower eyelid reveals many fairly typical superficial squamous epithelial cells with small nuclei. This is suggestive of a benign or low-grade epithelial proliferation such as a papilloma. Stippling and granules can sometimes be seen in the cytoplasm of these epithelial cells. In young dogs this lesion may spontaneously regress if not secondary to a persistent source of irritation. Removal of enlarging lesions, with biopsy evaluation, is recommended to ensure that this is not an emerging squamous cell carcinoma. In cats benign lesions are uncommon, and early removal is suggested. On occasion the epithelial cells will be pigmented, and melanoma can be added to the differential list.

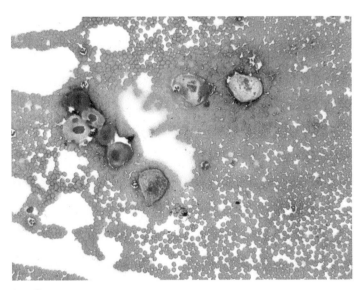

Figure 2.17 Canine conjunctival papilloma FNA. 10x.

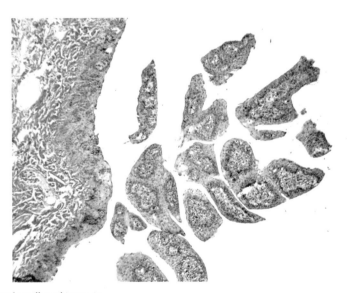

Figure 2.18 Canine conjunctival papilloma biopsy. 4x.

Figure 2.18 shows a canine conjunctival papilloma. A small papillary mass was removed from the anterior conjunctival surface of the right nictitans of a 6-year-old neutered male Golden Retriever. In the area of the mass the conjunctiva is comprised of multilayered well-differentiated poorly keratinized stratified squamous epithelium. The mass is micronodular to papillary and unevenly pigmented. It rises above the conjunctival surface and is on a short narrow stalk. It is lined by well-differentiated poorly keratinized stratified squamous epithelium, and no koilocytes (swollen epithelial cells with gray cytoplasm-viral cytopathic effects) were seen after a moderate search, so the papilloma is presumed to be nonviral and was probably caused by chronic irritation. The mass had a narrow base and appears resected. Nonviral conjunctival papillomas can be solitary or multicentric, and they are occasionally bilateral. Complete resection is usually curative for individual nonviral canine conjunctival papillomas.

Squamous cell carcinoma
Figure 2.19 shows feline squamous cell carcinoma. This scraping of a conjunctival lesion on the eyelid of an aged neutered male Domestic Short-hair cat revealed epithelial cells with moderate anisokaryosis and nuclear sizes discordant with the amount of cytoplasm and degree of cytoplasmic basophilia, suggesting a neoplastic proliferation. Chronic inflammation may result in epithelial atypia, and there are neutrophils closely associated with the atypical cells, but

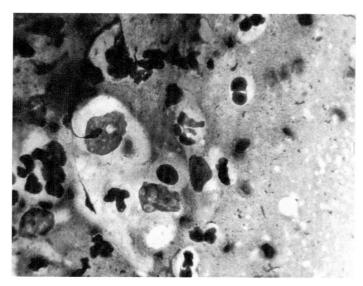

Figure 2.19 Feline squamous cell carcinoma FNA. 50x.

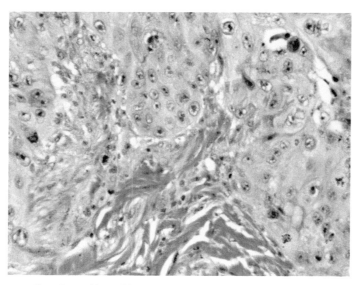

Figure 2.20 Feline ocular squamous cell carcinoma biopsy. 20x.

there is no evidence of infectious agents. It is presumed that the inflammation is a result of neoplasia. This lesion is likely to be a squamous cell carcinoma, and histologic evaluation is recommended.

Figure 2.20 shows a feline ocular squamous cell carcinoma. A 15-year-old spayed female Domestic Shorthair cat developed pink proliferative tissue at the ventral lateral limbus of the left eye. A globe with 0.8-cm tan smooth mass bulging from one edge of the cornea was submitted. The cornea had an adjacent opaque bulge. One cross section through the globe and mass was submitted for histopathology. A very poorly circumscribed infiltrative mass involving the conjunctiva and the cornea on one side of the section is comprised of pleomorphic medium to large polygonal epithelial cells with moderate variation in cell and nuclear size, scant to moderate eosinophilic cytoplasm, and numerous mitotic figures, some of them abnormal. Individual pigmented cells and pigment-laden macrophages are embedded in the stroma of this poorly circumscribed infiltrative mass. The corneal epithelium is mildly to moderately dysplastic in most areas, and there are some additional small nodules of infiltrative neoplastic squamous epithelium in the cornea on the opposite side of the globe, accompanied by chronic interstitial inflammation. Definitive intralymphatic embolization was not recognized at the level examined. This neoplasm is a squamous cell carcinoma, and it was infiltrative and also multicentric. In felines these tumors are sometimes multifocal, as in this case. Palpebral conjunctiva is a common site of origin. Actinic damage is a predisposing factor. Eventual metastasis to draining lymph nodes can occur.

Hemangiosarcoma

Figure 2.21 shows a feline hemangiosarcoma. Aspirate of a dark conjunctival mass reveals moderate to dense blood with platelet clumps indicative of acute hemorrhage, increased neutrophils, and scattered epithelioid cells occasionally demonstrating marked anisokaryosis (arrow), large nucleoli, cytoplasmic basophilia, and an eosinophilic tinged border (amphophilia). The large cells are presumed to be neoplastic endothelial cells, and the diagnosis is vascular tumor, presumptive hemangiosarcoma. Biopsy is recommended for definitive diagnosis as other sarcomas may have this cytologic appearance.

Figure 2.22 shows a biopsy of a feline conjunctival hemangiosarcoma. The left eye of a 12-year-old neutered male Domestic Shorthair cat had a red vascular mass 6 × 6 × 3 mm involving the ventral cornea and conjunctiva. The enucleated globe was submitted with an ill-defined micronodular tan mass 1.5 × 1.2 × 0.5 cm on the outside of the globe involving the cornea and sclera. Two sections through the globe and the external mass were processed. The mass appeared completely resected grossly. This mass is comprised by endothelial cells that line capillary and more cavernous blood-filled spaces. Most cells are mononuclear. Occasional cells have more than one nucleus. Occasional mitoses were found in this cell population (<1/10 HPF). The mass in the conjunctiva bulged and was multilobular, while the portion that infiltrated the superficial cornea was a thickened plaque. This mass is a hemangiosarcoma. It had

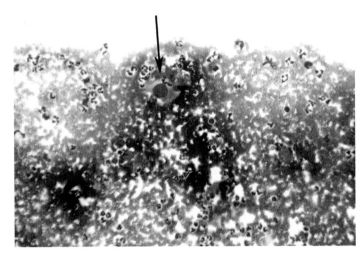

Figure 2.21 Feline hemangiosarcoma FNA. 10x.

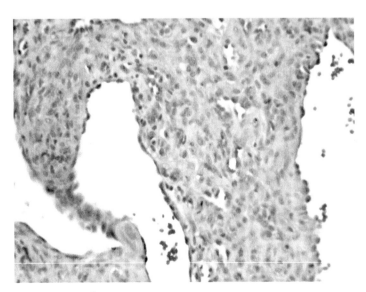

Figure 2.22 Feline conjunctival hemangiosarcoma biopsy. 20x.

infiltrated the cornea, so enucleation was the treatment of choice in this case. These tumors are often slow to metastasize, and timely enucleation can be curative. Note that in many species these tumors tend to arise in areas of chronic actinic damage, and they may be multiple. Periodic rechecks of the other eye were recommended, and the owner was advised that this patient should be protected from the sun.

Melanoma

Figure 2.23 shows a canine conjunctival melanoma. There is a population of epithelioid cells with dense cytoplasmic melanin granules and what appears to be mild anisokaryosis. The background is filled with rod-shaped melanin granules. The individual appearance of the granules within the cytoplasm suggests that these cells are well-differentiated melanocytes rather than melanophages.

Figure 2.24 shows a biopsy of a canine conjunctival melanoma. A small pigmented conjunctival mass in the region of the lateral canthus of the right eye was removed from a 6-year-old neutered male Golden Retriever. It was heavily pigmented in most areas but unpigmented in a few areas. It was multilobular, involving the mucosa and submucosa with slight encroachment on an underlying meibomian gland lobule. The mass was in the conjunctiva near the

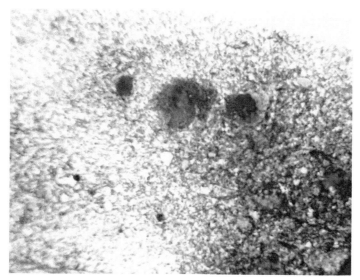

Figure 2.23 Canine conjunctival melanoma FNA. 50x.

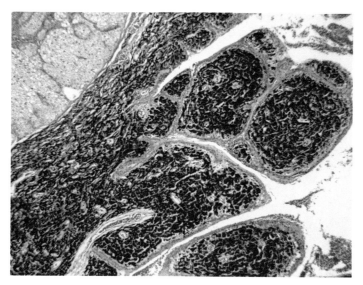

Figure 2.24 Canine conjunctival melanoma biopsy. 4x.

mucocutaneous junction. It was lined by somewhat attenuated poorly keratinized stratified squamous epithelium with junctional activity in some areas. About 2/3 of the mass was comprised of sheets and vague coalescing aggregates of small to medium heavily pigmented melanocytic cells with scattered individual heavily pigmented melanophages. In one area the cells were poorly pigmented and more spindloid. All nuclei were fairly regular, small, and usually mononuclear, and no mitoses were seen after a moderate search of the unpigmented area. The mass extended focally into the deep margin in one area within the conjunctiva as the convoluted specimen was cut. Other identifiable margins were clean. This pigmented conjunctival mass is a melanoma. The cells comprising it had a low mitotic rate (accurate MI calculation hampered by heavy pigmentation), and the cells appear well differentiated. The conjunctiva of the third eyelid is a relatively common site for melanomas in canines, and these tumors are often cytologically and behaviorally malignant with a fairly high rate of recurrence, although metastasis to distant sites is not often reported. Fairly careful follow-up of the surgical site and draining lymph nodes was advised.

Eyelid masses

Eyelid masses can be masked by hair until they become large or ulcerated. Meibomian gland hyperplasia and adenomas are common. Apocrine glands of the eyelid may also proliferate and form masses at the mucosal margin or in the haired skin. Spindle cell tumors may arise from nerves, muscles, and stromal elements around the eye. Cytologic exam can allow the clinician to decide if surgical removal is urgent and if margins must be large.

Meibomian gland adenoma

Figure 2.25 shows a canine meibomian gland adenoma. Aspiration of an eyelid mass on the upper lid of a female Mastiff revealed clusters of plump epithelioid cells with abundant finely vacuolated cytoplasm, small nuclei, and a few adjacent basaloid cells in a background of blood. This tumor type is usually low grade and can be excised with small margins, but biopsy confirmation is recommended to confirm the suspected tumor type.

Figure 2.26 shows a biopsy of a canine meibomian adenoma. A right upper eyelid mass was submitted from an 11-year-old spayed female Wireaired Pointer that had been slowly enlarging and bleeding periodically. The mass is comprised of multiple lobules of proliferating basaloid cells with multifocal sebaceous differentiation. Scattered here and there are squamous-lined ducts. The stroma is somewhat fibrotic and inflamed. The mass was mostly on the conjunctival side of the biopsy. The surface was focally eroded to ulcerated. Margins on the sections examined were clean. This is a benign neoplasm, which may be multifocal and bilateral. Complete resection is usually curative for such individual nodules.

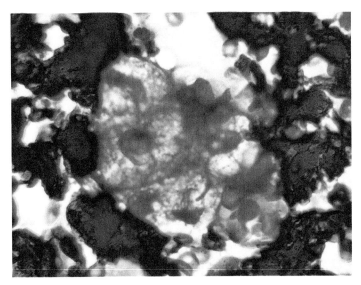

Figure 2.25 Canine meibomian gland adenoma FNA. 40x.

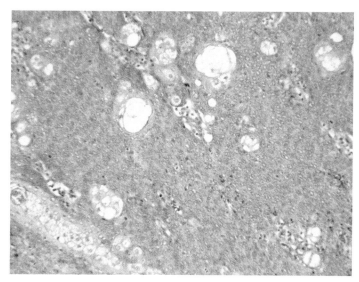

Figure 2.26 Canine meibomian adenoma biopsy. 10x.

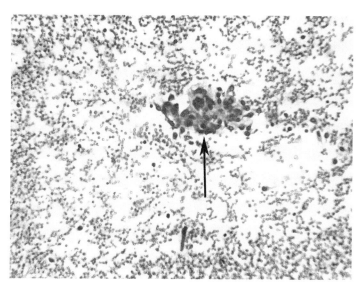

Figure 2.27 Canine spindle cell tumor FNA. 50x.

Spindle cell tumor

Figure 2.27 shows a canine spindle cell tumor. Aspirate of a periorbital mass on a male Terrier mix reveals clusters of spindle cells (arrow) with wispy pale cytoplasm, oblong nuclei, and mild to rare moderate anisokaryosis in a background of moderate blood. These cells are typical of mid- to high-grade spindle cell tumors arising from fibroblasts, muscles, nerves, and vascular walls and are indistinguishable by cytological exam. Granulation tissue can sometimes yield pleomorphic spindle cells on FNA due to the proliferation of reactive blood vessels and fibroblasts during healing, but large clumps of cells would be more supportive of neoplasia. Biopsy is recommended for a more definitive diagnosis.

Figure 2.28 shows canine spindle cell sarcoma. A clinical history was not provided. A whole eye was submitted. It was a globe with an adjacent previously partially incised tan-brown micronodular mass possibly representing the third eyelid. The globe was compressed but did not appear to have been deeply invaded by the mass. One representative section though the mass with a portion of adjacent globe was submitted for histologic examination. This is a multilobular mass of neoplastic polygonal and plump spindle cells. These cells are organized in vague interlacing bundles. Most areas are cellular with scant stroma. The cells have oval to elongated nuclei with one or two nucleoli. Mitoses occurred in low numbers. MI = 0/10 HPF. Occasional multinucleated cells were noted. Cytoplasm is generally eosinophilic and

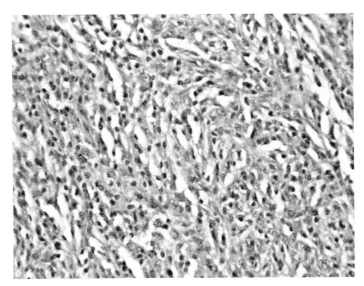

Figure 2.28 Canine spindle cell sarcoma biopsy. 20x.

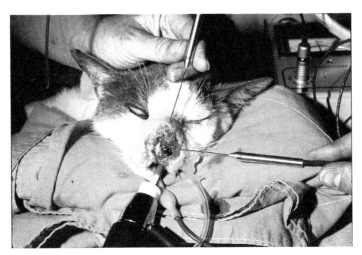

Figure 2.29 Gross photograph of an ulcerative lesion on the nose of a cat. (Courtesy of the College of Veterinary Medicine, University of Florida, Gainesville, FL.)

streaming with indistinct borders. The spindle cell tumors are difficult to differentiate by light microscopy. The most common differentials include fibrosarcoma, canine hemangiopericytoma, and tumors of nerve or nerve sheath origin (neurofibroma, neurofibrosarcoma, schwannoma). Nerve sheath origin was suspected in this case because of cytologic features and proliferative pattern. However, all of these tumors are slow to metastasize but are famous for local recurrence. Therefore, radical resection and careful follow-up are usually recommended.

Lesions of the oral and nasal mucosal epithelium

Lesions on the external nose are often noticed early in the course of the disease, but occasionally they manifest in an intermittent manner (eosinophilic ulcer, mast cell tumor). If they arise from internal structures, there may be no obvious signs until nasal hemorrhage occurs.

Figure 2.29 shows gross presentation of an ulcerative lesion on the nose of a cat. Inflammatory and neoplastic processes can result in marked tissue destruction over time.

Eosinophilic inflammation

Figure 2.30 shows canine dorsal nose eosinophilic inflammation. Dogs and cats can have lesions containing large populations of eosinophils (arrowheads). If more than 25% of the inflammatory leukocytes from an impression or scrape of an ulcerated mass are eosinophils, in the face of a normal peripheral blood eosinophil count, eosinophilic inflammation is recognized. There can be pools of eosinophil granules accumulated after degeneration of large numbers of eosinophils. Scattered neutrophils and bacteria can be seen at the surface. There are often metabolically active superficial squamous epithelial cells as a result of chronic re-epithelialization. Etiologies can include fungal infection, insect bites, a foreign body response secondary to penetrating injury, a familial predilection, autoimmune disease, drug reaction, or a systemic hypersensitivity response to inhaled, dietary, or parasitic antigens. In cats this lesion can be a result of herpesvirus infection in addition to the previously listed etiologies, and can appear superficial and ulcerated (indolent ulcer) or deep and nodular (eosinophilic granuloma).

Figure 2.31 shows a biopsy of a canine eosinophilic granuloma on the dorsal nose. This adult female Husky had a focally ulcerated and deep multilobular mass on the dorsal nose. Infectious agents were not seen with routine stains. There is an increased incidence in this breed. There was intermittent response to immunosuppressive therapy.

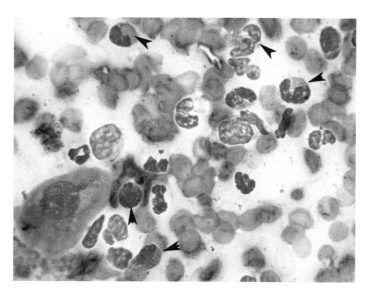

Figure 2.30 Canine dorsal nose eosinophilic inflammation impression. 50x.

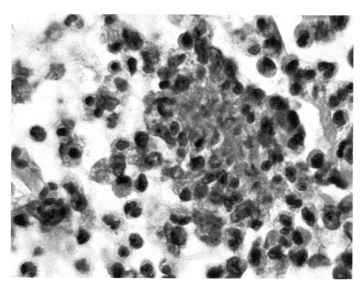

Figure 2.31 Canine eosinophilic granuloma on dorsal nose biopsy. 40x.

Dogs and cats with inflammatory lesions of the oral mucosa may present with clinical signs of drooling, halitosis, or inability to eat. Physical exam may reveal a diffuse and variably ulcerated swelling of the oral mucous membranes. Deep scraping may yield diagnostic cell populations. Cytologic exam may reveal inflammatory leukocytes with greater than 25% eosinophils, suggesting eosinophilic inflammation. Eosinophilic ulcer would be the tentative diagnosis, but biopsy is recommended to exclude a neoplastic etiology. Ulcerated mucosal epithelium with submucosal dense infiltrates of eosinophils around foci of collagen necrosis and free eosinophil granules is the hallmark of oral eosinophilic ulcer (indolent ulcer, rodent ulcer).

Lymphoplasmacellular inflammation

Figure 2.32 shows feline lymphoplasmacellular stomatitis from scraping. Scraping or aspirating a diffuse gingival lesion may yield a dense mixed population of small lymphocytes and plasma cells. This mixed population in this adult female Persian is likely a response to antigenic stimulation such as viral infection or dental disease. Impression smear is likely to yield only superficial debris.

Figure 2.33 shows feline lymphoplasmacellular stomatitis. Diffuse infiltrates of lymphocytes and plasma cells in this 5-year-old feline immunodeficiency virus positive Domestic Shorthair cat form nodular, sometimes ulcerated,

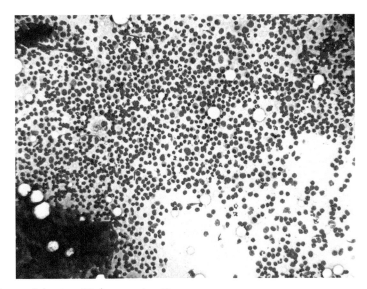

Figure 2.32 Feline lymphoplasmacellular stomatitis from scraping. 10x.

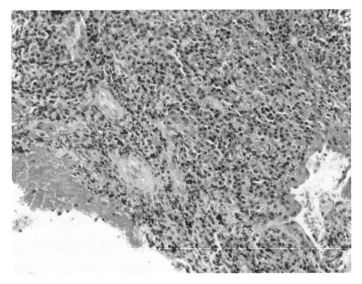

Figure 2.33 Feline lymphoplasmacellular stomatitis biopsy. 10x.

proliferations in the gingival and oral submucosa. Periodontal disease can be the cause or the result of this intense inflammation. Etiologies include traumatic injury, systemic diseases that cause chronic immunosuppression or vasculitis, renal disease, or if the lesion is focal, leaking or inflamed salivary or submucosal glands.

Lymphosarcoma

Figure 2.34 shows feline mucocutaneous lymphosarcoma. Cytologic evaluation of a mucosal swab from a 10-year-old neutered male Birman cat reveals a dense population of lymphocytes, larger than accompanying neutrophils, with multiple nucleoli and basophilic cytoplasm. These cells are monomorphic in appearance, suggesting derivation from a common ancestor, which is a prerequisite of clonality, and exhibit the basophilic metabolically active cytoplasm that can be seen with the uncontrolled proliferation of a high-grade lymphoid neoplasm. Clonality can be confirmed by polymerase chain reaction (PCR) of antigen receptor site rearrangements (PARR) performed on cells taken from this stained slide or flow cytometry of a freshly collected sample.

Figure 2.35 shows feline nasal turbinate with mucocutaneous lymphosarcoma. This 3-year-old female Domestic Shorthair presented with nasal discharge. The biopsy revealed expansion of the submucosa of the nasal turbinate by an abnormally dense population of round cells larger than the accompanying neutrophils and eosinophils, with occasional

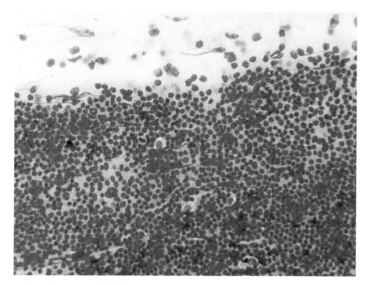

Figure 2.34 Feline mucocutaneous lymphosarcoma FNA. 10x.

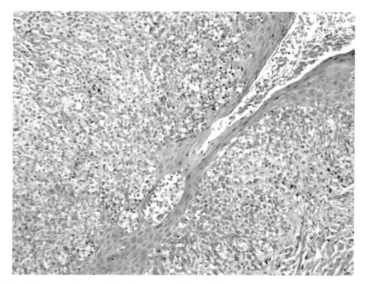

Figure 2.35 Feline nasal turbinate with mucocutaneous lymphosarcoma biopsy. 10x.

invasion into the underlying bone and overlying epithelial layer. This population of round cells is typical of lymphoid neoplasia and could be confirmed and classified as to T- or B-cell origin by immunohistochemistry.

Epulis

Figure 2.36 shows a canine epulis. This focal, glistening pink mass is most likely an epulis (peripheral odontogenic fibroma), but FNA can be a useful early tool to evaluate the cell population for benign or malignant cellular features. This helps the surgeon determine the appropriate margin width.

Acanthomatous epulis

Figure 2.37 shows a canine epulis. Aspirate of a gingival mass at the lower right incisor of an adult male Boxer reveals small sheets of well-differentiated superficial squamous epithelium (arrowhead) with occasional slender spindle cells in a background that often includes neutrophils, cellular debris, and sometimes mixed oral bacteria. Scant eosinophilic material (arrow) is suggestive of stromal matrix or osteoid. This poorly cellular population is suggestive of an epulis.

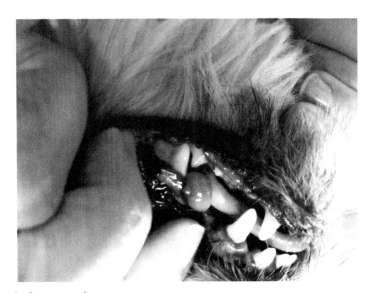

Figure 2.36 Clinical photograph of a canine epulis.

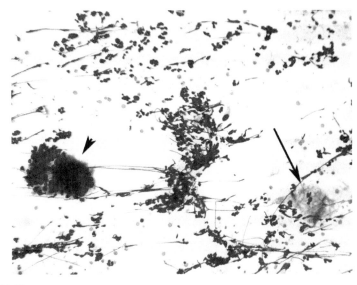

Figure 2.37 Canine epulis FNA. 10x.

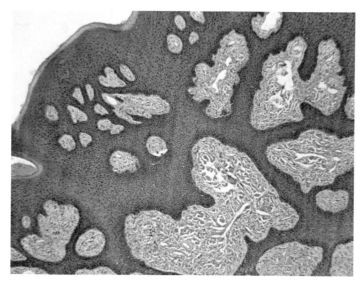

Figure 2.38 Canine fibromatous epulis (peripheral odontogenic fibroma), biopsy. 4x.

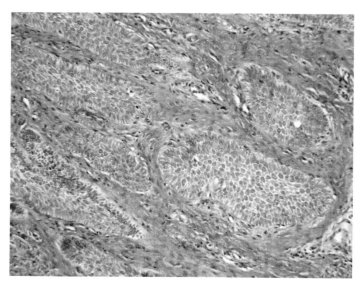

Figure 2.39 Canine acanthomatous epulis (acanthomatous ameloblastoma), biopsy. 10x.

Figure 2.38 shows a canine fibromatous epulis. A neutered male Bloodhound of unknown age had a 2-cm pedunculated gingival mass covering the upper left first and second incisors and a similar mass over the upper right first incisor. Representative sections of each were submitted. The irregular surface is covered by thick well-differentiated stratified squamous epithelium with epitheliomatous hyperplasia in the underlying cellular and well-vascularized dense fibrous connective tissue stroma. There are additional islands of smaller epithelial cells with intercellular bridges but without peripheral palisading. Both lesions extended into the margins as the convoluted specimens were cut. Epulides are considered benign, but they are frequently multiple, and they can recur after resection.

Figure 2.39 shows a canine acanthomatous epulis. This is another example of the gingival mass described above with more dramatic peripheral palisading around the borders of the infiltrating epithelial trabeculae.

Ossifying epulis

Figure 2.40 shows a canine ossifying epulis. This aspirate of an oral mass from an 8-year-old male neutered Siberian Husky mix dog revealed clusters of well-differentiated superficial mucosal epithelium (arrowhead) with small nuclei adjacent to eosinophilic amorphous material compatible with bone matrix or osteoid (arrow). An ossifying epulis is suspected, but biopsy is recommended to exclude a well-differentiated squamous cell carcinoma invading bone.

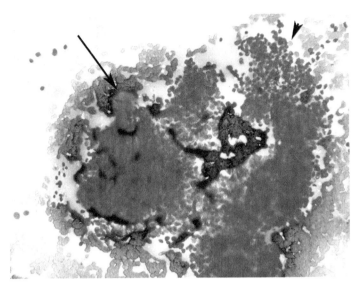

Figure 2.40 Canine ossifying epulis FNA. 10x.

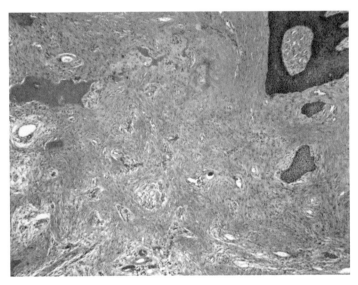

Figure 2.41 Canine ossifying epulis (ossifying peripheral odontogenic fibroma), biopsy. 4x.

Figure 2.41 shows a canine ossifying epulis. A 6-year-old spayed female Retriever Cross had an epulis-like mass over a tooth. It was similar to the fibromatous epulis described above, but the stroma also contained osteoid deposits and fragments of immature bone. Lymphocytes and plasma cells followed the basement membrane of the surface epithelium in one area, which was adjacent to the tooth. The lesion extended into the margins. Chronic epulides tend to ossify.

Viral papilloma

Figure 2.42 shows a canine oral papilloma scraping. Cytologic exam of cells scraped from an oral mass in a 6-month-old Labradoodle reveals epithelial cells with nuclei about the size of a neutrophil, occasional moderate anisokaryosis but with moderately dense chromatin and no detectable nucleoli. There is abundant pale to amphophilic cytoplasm with occasional metachromatic granules suggestive of keratinizing superficial squamous cells. Rare dense purple cytoplasmic structures may be viral inclusions, but overlying round erythrocytes can mimic this feature.

Figure 2.43 shows canine oral papilloma. Biopsy of an oral mass from a 1-year-old male Husky dog revealed papillary fronds of hyperkeratotic squamous epithelium over a fibrous stroma. Eosinophilic material in the cytoplasm of some cells is suggestive of viral inclusions. Papilloma virus is known to produce generally benign epithelial proliferations,

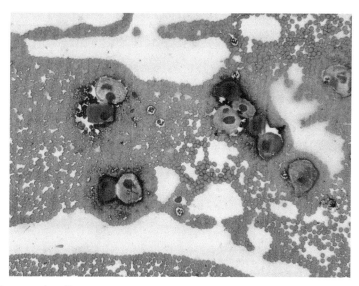

Figure 2.42 Canine oral papilloma scraping. 10x.

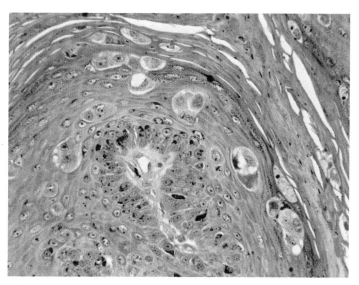

Figure 2.43 Canine oral papilloma biopsy. 20x.

and a strong immune system will usually cause regression with time. A weak immune response or immunosuppression can lead to multiple lesions, recurrent lesions, and on rare occasion, malignant transformation. Stromal invasion is not seen in this biopsy, and often complete excision is curative.

Squamous cell carcinoma

Figure 2.44 shows feline oral squamous cell carcinoma FNA. There are clusters of epithelial cells with moderate aniso-karyosis and a cell with two nuclei that are molded against each other (arrowhead). There are recognizable nucleoli in cells with abundant, pale, keratinizing cytoplasm (as evidenced by scattered small vacuoles and pale eosinophilic granules) whose nuclei should be shrinking and becoming pyknotic and metabolically inactive. Neutrophils are sometimes seen in the cytoplasm of the neoplastic epithelial cells (arrow).

Figure 2.45 shows a feline mandibular squamous cell carcinoma biopsy. A portion of the right mandible with a tumor was removed from a 14-year-old neutered male Domestic Shorthair cat. The specimen was decalcified, and one cross section through a thickened area was processed. The mass was poorly circumscribed and infiltrative, and the stroma was scirrhous. The neoplasm is comprised of pleomorphic enlarged squamous epithelial cells that form irregular nodules and infiltrative trabeculae. Central keratinization, dyskeratosis, and inflamed keratin pearls were noted.

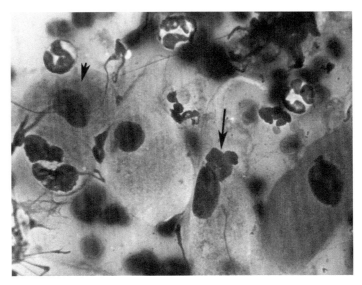

Figure 2.44 Feline oral squamous cell carcinoma FNA. 50x.

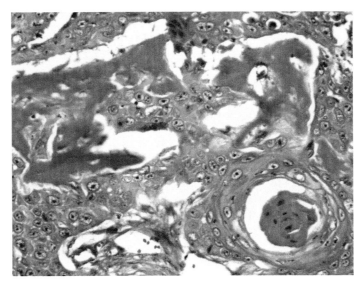

Figure 2.45 Feline mandibular squamous cell carcinoma biopsy. 20x.

The involved bone is largely destroyed. Definitive intralymphatic/intravascular embolization was not seen at the levels examined, and the deep margin on the central representative section was clean. Feline oral tumors are usually malignant, and squamous cell carcinoma is a common gingival neoplasm in cats. Squamous cell carcinomas can also develop in the feline tongue and at various other sites within the oral cavity. Even if completely resected, these tumors can metastasize via lymphatics to regional mandibular and retropharyngeal lymph nodes. The tumors can also recur at the site of mandibulectomy, so careful follow-up is usually advised.

Melanoma

Figure 2.46 shows canine oral melanoma. Aspirate of a variably dark to fleshy mass from the mouth of a 6-year-old Rottweiler dog reveals pleomorphic spindloid to epithelioid cells with marked anisokaryosis, prominent multiple nucleoli, variably basophilic cytoplasm, and rare cells with scant melanin granules. This degree of nuclear and cytoplasmic pleomorphism is typical of aggressive melanomas, and it may be difficult to find cells with the diagnostic cytoplasmic melanin granules without resorting to the 100x oil lens.

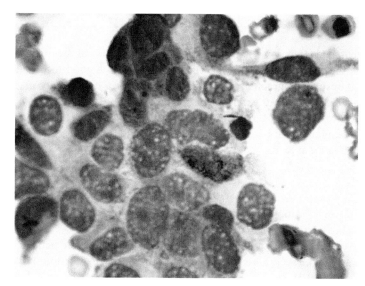

Figure 2.46 Canine oral melanoma FNA. 50x.

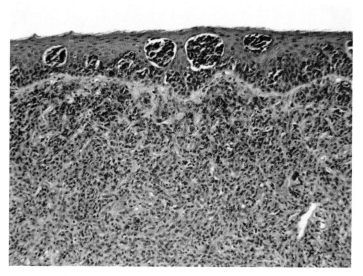

Figure 2.47 Canine oral melanoma biopsy. 10x.

Figure 2.47 shows a canine oral melanoma. A 14-1/2-year-old neutered male Standard Poodle was presented for a recurrent oral buccal mucosal melanoma. A glabrous specimen with an ill-defined raised pigmented area was submitted, along with an extra marginal piece. This is a melanoma of epithelioid cell type that involved the mucosa and submucosa, and junctional activity extended peripheral to the mass on both sides of the primary specimen. The mass has a scant to moderate fibrovascular stroma, and it is comprised of vague coalescing aggregates of mildly pleomorphic, often rather poorly pigmented melanocytic cells with mild variation in cell and nuclear size, and scattered cells have more than one nucleus. MI = 2/10 HPF. Most of the pigmented cells are superficial in the lesion. Large aggregates of pigmented neoplastic melanocytic cells are embedded in the overlying epithelium, and these cellular islands extended peripheral to the primary plaque-like lesion. Margins were clean. Deep margin = 3.5 mm in the center. Narrowest lateral margin from the intra-epithelial neoplastic cellular islands = 1.5 mm. An additional portion of mucosa from the rostral aspect had no histologic evidence of neoplasia. However, periodic rechecks of this surgical site and draining lymph nodes were advised. Canine oral melanomas are usually malignant, and many of them recur locally. They spread readily to draining lymph nodes and the lungs, as well.

Nasal cavity tumors

Masses within the nasal cavity are often not discovered until late in the course of the disease when there is a nosebleed or significant distortion of the face. Traumatic catheterization or FNA is a good technique to obtain a preliminary diagnosis before taking a biopsy. Radiographs can be useful to look for a nasal cavity mass or an area of bone lysis suitable for biopsy if there is not an obvious external mass. Other imaging modalities such as computed tomography (CT) or magnetic resonance imaging (MRI) may be necessary if a lesion is not identified by preliminary radiographs. Complete surgical excision of nasal tumors can be difficult, and consultation with a specialist is recommended for formulation of an appropriate treatment plan.

Adenocarcinoma

Figure 2.48 shows feline nasal adenocarcinoma. Aspiration of a frontal sinus swelling on a 10-year-old spayed female Domestic Shorthair cat revealed clumps of epithelioid cells with marked anisokaryosis, prominent nucleoli and basophilic cytoplasm typical of nasal adenocarcinoma.

Figure 2.49 shows a biopsy of a feline frontal sinus adenocarcinoma. A 17-year-old neutered male Domestic Shorthair cat developed a swelling between the eyes. Bone was involved, with a suspected communication with the frontal sinus.

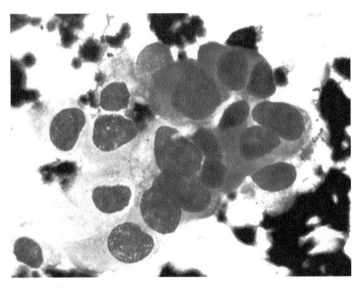

Figure 2.48 Feline nasal adenocarcinoma FNA. 50x.

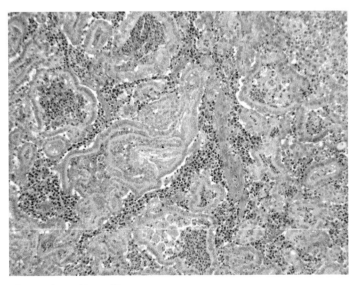

Figure 2.49 Feline frontal sinus adenocarcinoma biopsy. 10x.

Punch biopsies were submitted. The mass was an inflamed multilobular epithelial neoplasm. It is comprised of medium-sized polygonal, cuboidal, and columnar epithelial cells that form acini and slightly dilated tubules or glands. Thus, the swelling was apparently due to a neoplasm that developed in the mucosal glands of the frontal sinus. Nasal and sinus carcinomas are locally aggressive, and they are often difficult to completely resect. Metastatic potential is low. These tumors can spread via lymphatics, but this usually occurs late in the course of the disease.

Chondrosarcoma

Figure 2.50 shows a canine nasal chondrosarcoma. Aspirate of a firm nasal swelling on an adult neutered male Beagle revealed many epithelioid cells with moderate anisokaryosis, occasional binucleate (arrowhead) and trinucleate cells (arrow), and moderate amphophilic cytoplasm in a metachromatic matrix. This population is typical of a cartilage or bone-producing tumor. The pleomorphic nuclei suggest an aggressive tumor.

Figure 2.51 shows a canine nasal chondrosarcoma biopsy. A 9-year-old neutered male Labrador Retriever had a history of recurrent hemorrhagic right nasal discharge. Radiographs showed a loss of turbinate detail on the right side and an area of calcification and increased density in the right nasal sinus. Three biopsies were submitted. One revealed chronic sinusitis with moderate numbers of hemosiderin-laden macrophages. The two more solid specimens were comprised of lobules of chondrocytes of greatly varied cell and nuclear size. The amount of cartilaginous matrix varied.

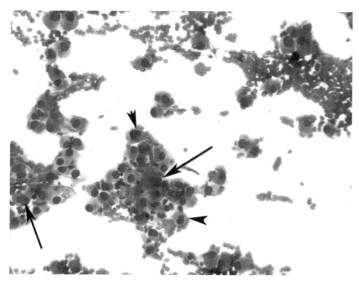

Figure 2.50 Canine nasal chondrosarcoma FNA. 10x.

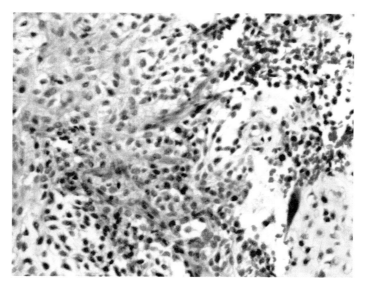

Figure 2.51 Canine nasal chondrosarcoma biopsy. 20x.

No mitoses were seen in the solid cellular cartilaginous areas, but some cells have more than one nucleus. Cartilaginous tumors in the nasal sinuses are locally aggressive and are likely to recur if not widely resected, which is often not possible. However, they are usually slow to metastasize.

Mass lesions of the canine and feline muzzle skin

Raised, circumscribed, often ulcerated lesions of the haired skin of the face are commonly seen lesions in the dog, and this condition is sometimes seen in the cat. FNA is useful to obtain a preliminary diagnosis because this clinical presentation is similar for many different types of lesions ranging from granulomas to benign cysts to neoplasms such as mast cell tumor.

Figure 2.52 shows an adult dog presenting with an ulcerated and bleeding mass. It is very difficult to reliably identify the type of lesion by gross evaluation. FNA will help to evaluate the components of the lesion so appropriate medical or surgical therapy can be chosen. If this is a mast cell tumor it would be prudent to obtain wider margins than if this is a sebaceous gland tumor.

Sebaceous gland nodular hyperplasia

Figure 2.53 shows a canine sebaceous gland proliferation. Aspirate of a raised ulcerated mass on an aged spayed female mixed breed dog yields clumps of sebaceous gland epithelium. Biopsy is necessary to determine if the proliferation is due to hyperplasia or neoplasia.

Figure 2.54 shows a biopsy of a canine nodular sebaceous gland hyperplasia. A 7-year-old spayed female Cocker Spaniel had a mass removed from the left ventral neck. The specimen contains a mass composed of multilobular proliferations of well-differentiated sebaceous glands organized around somewhat dilated squamous lined ducts. A central branching duct lined by stratified squamous epithelium was dilated. Leakage of sebum had incited a foreign body response peripheral to

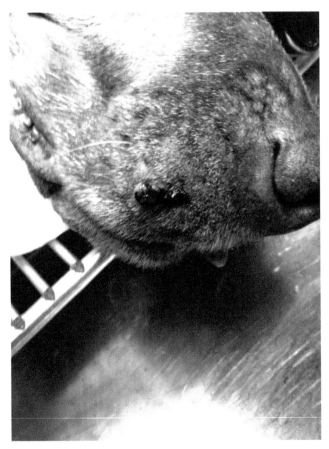

Figure 2.52 A photograph of an adult dog with an ulcerated and bleeding muzzle mass.

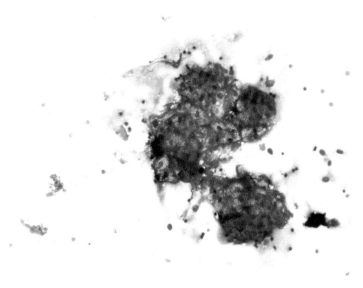

Figure 2.53 Canine sebaceous gland proliferation FNA. 10x.

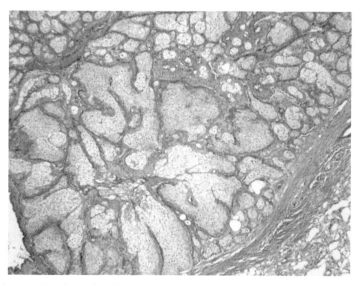

Figure 2.54 Canine nodular sebaceous gland hyperplasia biopsy. 4x.

the primary mass. Margins were clean. This is a benign lesion, which is frequently multifocal. Inflammation is a common complication. There is an increased incidence of abnormal sebaceous gland proliferations in Cocker Spaniels.

Sebaceous gland adenoma

Figure 2.55 shows a canine sebaceous adenoma biopsy. A 9-year-old neutered male Jack Russell Terrier had an oozing irritated mass on the neck. A representative section was examined. This mass is comprised of multiple lobules of proliferating basaloid cells with frequent sebaceous differentiation. Scattered here and there were squamous-lined ducts. The stroma was somewhat fibrotic and inflamed. The surface was ulcerated and covered with serous exudate. Margins on the section were clean. Surgical resection is usually curative. This tumor has more basaloid cells and less mature sebaceous cells than the focus of nodular sebaceous gland hyperplasia described in Figure 2.54.

Sebaceous epithelioma

Figure 2.56 shows a canine sebaceous epithelioma biopsy. There were multiple tumors above the right eye of a 10-year-old neutered male Cocker Spaniel. Part of the mass pictured is comprised of multiple lobules of proliferating basaloid cells with frequent sebaceous differentiation and small squamous-lined ducts. Most of the mass is comprised of multiple

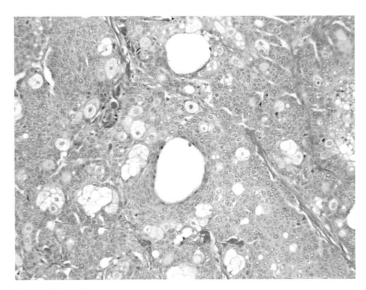

Figure 2.55 Canine sebaceous adenoma biopsy. 10x.

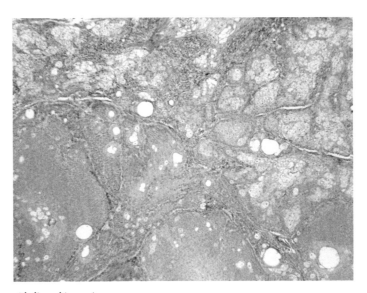

Figure 2.56 Canine sebaceous epithelioma biopsy. 4x.

lobules of proliferating basal cells with infrequent sebaceous differentiation, consistent with a sebaceous epithelioma. There was no evidence of stromal invasion or intralymphatic spread around the periphery, although there was some chronic inflammation. The surface was focally ulcerated, and there was an inflammatory crust on the surface at another site. Margins were clean. Surgical resection is the treatment of choice, and recurrence is unusual. However, these tumors are occasionally multiple. This section of tissue suggests a progression from a less aggressive lesion (adenomatous appearance in upper right) to a more aggressive lesion (epithelioma appearance in lower left). Malignant transformation with metastasis via lymphatics is rare. There seems to be an increased incidence of abnormal sebaceous gland proliferations in Cocker Spaniels.

Trichoblastoma (Basal cell tumor)

Figure 2.57 shows a feline trichoblastoma FNA. Aspirate of a muzzle mass may yield clusters of small basaloid epithelial cells with a few slender spindle cells in a background of scant blood. The small and monomorphic nature of the nuclei is suggestive of a low-grade adnexal tumor such as a trichoblastoma.

Figure 2.58 shows a feline trichoblastoma biopsy. A 4-year-old neutered male Maine Coon cat developed a pink raised hairless mass on the right upper lip near the whiskers. The mass was bisected and totally submitted as two

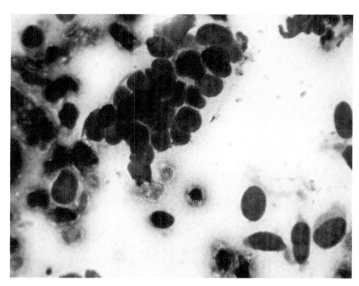

Figure 2.57 Feline trichoblastoma (basal cell tumor) FNA. 50x.

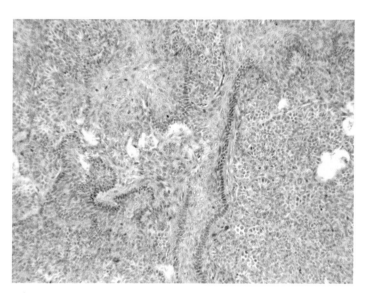

Figure 2.58 Feline trichoblastoma biopsy. 10x.

sections in one cassette. The mass was circumscribed but not encapsulated, and it had a moderate fibrous connective tissue stroma. It was comprised of thick anastomosing trabeculae of basaloid epithelial cells with peripheral palisading. Mitoses were seen at a rate of <1/HPF. Stromal invasion and intralymphatic spread were not recognized along the periphery, but the mass extended into the deep cauterized margin. Cauterized lateral skin margins were clean but narrow. This is a benign neoplasm of hair follicle origin currently called a trichoblastoma, trabecular type (previously called basal cell tumor.) These tumors generally do not metastasize, but occasionally they are multiple. The trabecular type usually occurs in cats. They can recur if not completely resected.

Figure 2.59 shows a canine trichoblastoma biopsy. A 2-cm round skin mass was removed from the left caudal commissure of the mouth of a 4-year-old Soft Coated Wheaten Terrier. The mass had doubled in size in 2 months. A representative section was examined histologically. The mass is composed of coalescing islands and chains of basaloid epithelial cells separated by fibrovascular stroma. Mitoses were infrequent in many areas but occurred in moderate numbers in others. Margins were clean. This is a ribbon-type trichoblastoma (previously called basal cell tumor.) These tumors generally do not metastasize, but occasionally they are multiple. The ribbon type is common in canines. Complete resection is usually curative.

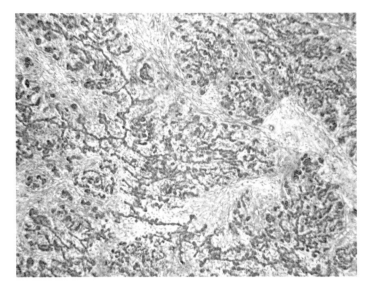

Figure 2.59 Canine trichoblastoma biopsy. 10x.

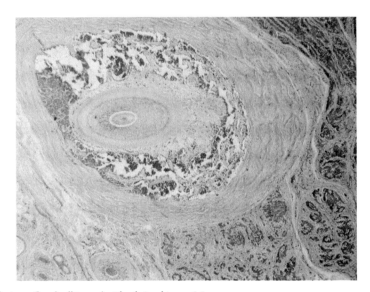

Figure 2.60 Canine trichoblastoma (basal cell tumor) with vibrissa biopsy. 2.5x.

Figure 2.60 shows a biopsy of a canine trichoblastoma with vibrissa. A muzzle mass from an adult male Boxer was submitted for biopsy, and adjacent to the ribbons of basaloid epithelial cells forming a trichoblastoma there is a normal vibrissa containing a whisker. This normal structure is sometimes presented for biopsy because it can have the appearance of a skin mass.

Mast cell tumor

Figure 2.61 shows a canine mast cell tumor FNA. Aspirate of a muzzle mass on a 5-year-old female Pug revealed many mast cells in a background of free mast cell granules. There is moderate nuclear pleomorphism, and this may be a high-grade tumor. Excisional biopsy is recommended for grading and evaluation of margins.

Figure 2.62 shows a biopsy of a canine mast cell tumor. An 8-year-old spayed female Catahoula Leopard Dog cross was presented for excision of multiple skin masses. The mass shown is from the right ventral neck. The specimen was skin and subcutis with a diffusing and rather poorly circumscribed infiltrate of variably granulated mast cells in sheets, vague small lobules, and narrow cords. There is mild variation in nuclear size. Cytoplasmic borders are distinct. Potential mitoses are infrequent. MI = 0/10 HPF, but scattered cells have double nuclei. Varied numbers of eosinophils accompany the mast cells. Ectatic apocrine sweat glands are entrapped in the fibrous stroma along the deep border

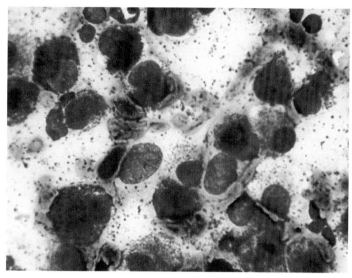

Figure 2.61 Canine mast cell tumor FNA. 50x.

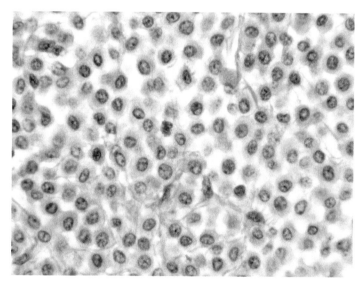

Figure 2.62 Canine mast cell tumor biopsy. 40x.

of the mass. This is a relatively common finding in canine cutaneous mast cell tumors. Margins were clean. Deep margin = 1.5 mm in the center. Narrowest lateral skin margin = 5 mm. The cells are still fairly well differentiated with a low mitotic rate, consistent with a grade 2 (three-level Patnaik system) or low-grade (two-tier grading system) canine mast cell tumor, and it appeared narrowly but completely resected. Nevertheless, behavior of these tumors is somewhat unpredictable. They are capable of local recurrence, multicentric appearance, and metastasis via lymphatics.

Plasma cell tumor

Figure 2.63 shows a canine plasmacytoma FNA. Aspiration of a raised skin mass on the muzzle of a 6-year-old male Cocker Spaniel reveals many round cells with round to pleomorphic and lobulated nuclei eccentrically placed in lightly basophilic cytoplasm. This tumor type can have an aggressive cytologic appearance due to the nuclear pleomorphism but is usually benign in behavior. Biopsy is suggested for confirmation of the tumor type.

Figure 2.64 shows a canine ear canal plasmacytoma biopsy. A neutered male canine of unknown breed was presented for an infected left ear. A lobulated tumor was removed from the left external ear canal. The mass is comprised of sheets of neoplastic round cells sometimes separated into vague nests by a fine fibrovascular stroma. The round cells are variable in size. Nuclei are round, oval, or irregular, and often hyperchromatic, with coarsely clumped chromatin.

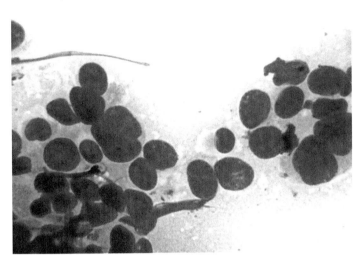

Figure 2.63 Canine plasmacytoma FNA. 50x.

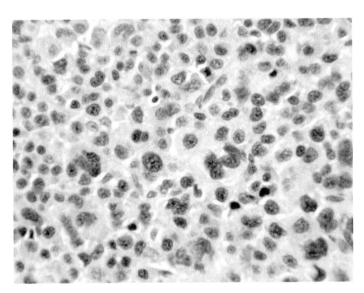

Figure 2.64 Canine ear canal plasmacytoma biopsy. 40x.

Cytoplasm is amphophilic and variable in amount, often with distinct cell borders. Mitoses occur in moderate numbers. The cells are agranular and unpigmented, and they look plasmacytoid. Scattered through the tumor are individual cells with large nuclei, double nuclei, multiple nuclei, or lobate nuclei. The mass was covered by thick well-differentiated stratified squamous epithelium with a moderate layer of orthokeratotic keratin on the surface. The mass extended into the margins of the convoluted specimen, as cut. These tumors are usually benign and solitary in dogs, in spite of their pleomorphic cytologic appearance. They can be found anywhere on the skin, and often are within the oral cavity, in or on the ears, or between the toes. These tumors can recur if not completely resected. There is an increased incidence in Cocker Spaniels, but any breed can be affected.

Mass lesions of the submandibular region

Submandibular masses, especially if bilateral, often originate from the submandibular lymph nodes or salivary glands. Aspiration of a submandibular mass can provide immediate detection of salivary gland or lymph node elements. If clearly neoplastic cells are seen, biopsy is indicated to identify the tumor type and give a prognosis. If the lesion is inflammatory, medical therapy may be the appropriate treatment.

Reactive lymph node

Figure 2.65 shows a feline reactive lymph node FNA. There is a mixed population of small to medium lymphocytes (lymphocytes smaller than or equal to the size of the neutrophils in the lower left of center) with scattered plasma cells, low numbers of blasts, and rare neutrophils. This mixed population, aspirated from a 2-year-old male Domestic Shorthair cat, is the hallmark of a reactive lymph node, but emerging well-differentiated lymphoid neoplasia cannot be excluded on the basis of a cytologic sample as only a small number of cells are seen, and there is no architectural arrangement to the cells. Submandibular lymph nodes are often very reactive, and if there is generalized lymphadenopathy another node such as a prescapular or popliteal node may be a better choice for aspiration.

Figure 2.66 shows a feline reactive lymph node biopsy. The architecture of a reactive node is demonstrated by this lymph node biopsy. There are cortical follicles composed of a round germinal center of large lymphocytes, macrophages, dendritic cells, and blasts, surrounded by a wall of small lymphocytes that give this area a darker appearance. Beyond the germinal center is a wall of plasma cells that fades into the medullary region with cords of small lymphocytes interspersed with sinusoids filled with plasma cells. Aspiration of this lymph node yields the mixed population of cells seen in Figure 2.65.

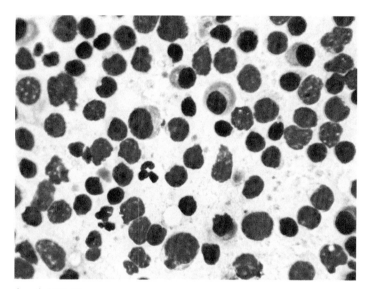

Figure 2.65 Feline reactive lymph node FNA. 50x.

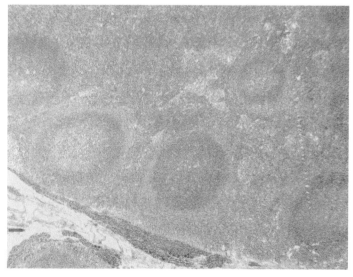

Figure 2.66 Feline reactive lymph node biopsy. 10x.

Malignant lymphoma

Figure 2.67 shows a canine malignant lymphoma (lymphosarcoma) FNA. Aspirate of an enlarged popliteal lymph node reveals a population of large round cells compatible with large lymphocytes, most of which are larger than the neutrophil near the top right of center. Some of the intact round cells demonstrate nucleoli (large arrows) identifying them as blasts, but many of the cells with multiple smaller "nucleoli" are broken and the structures that appear to be nucleoli may be artifact (arrowheads). Only cells with an intact cytoplasmic membrane should be used for cytologic interpretation (small arrows). This population is suggestive of high-grade lymphoma.

Figure 2.68 shows a biopsy of a canine malignant lymphoma of the mandibular lymph node. A 10-year-old neutered male King Charles Cavalier Spaniel was presented for generalized enlargement of lymph nodes. Multiple small biopsies were submitted, with insufficient fields for accurate evaluation of mitotic rate. The specimens were infiltrated by sheets of pleomorphic medium and large polygonal and round cells that appear lymphoid. These cells have nuclei 1.0 - 2.0 X red blood cell size. Many of the cells have a single prominent central nucleolus. Other cells have multiple smaller nucleoli. No normal lymphoid architecture was recognized in these multiple biopsies. The histology is consistent with malignant lymphoma, mixed immunoblastic, and diffuse large cell types. There was invasion of adjacent adipose and fibrovascular tissue. This is a multicentric disease, as described clinically in this case. Lymph nodes can be the first tissue involved, but this multicentric disease can eventually affect internal organs such as liver and spleen, bone marrow, and the peripheral blood.

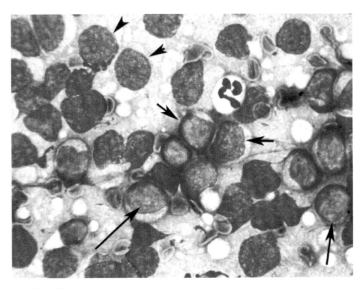

Figure 2.67 Canine lymphosarcoma FNA. 50x.

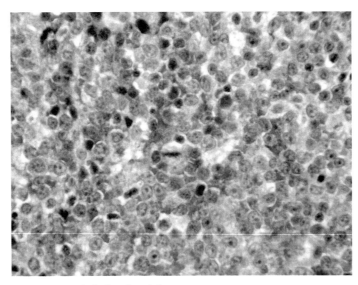

Figure 2.68 Canine malignant lymphoma, mandibular lymph node biopsy. 40x.

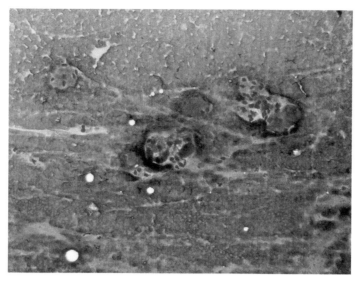

Figure 2.69 Normal canine salivary gland FNA. 10x.

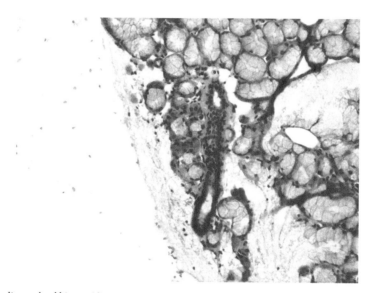

Figure 2.70 Normal canine salivary gland biopsy. 10x.

Normal salivary gland

Figure 2.69 shows a normal canine salivary gland FNA. This is an aspirate of a normal salivary gland with clusters of glandular epithelium (serous and mucous types) and smaller basaloid (ductular) epithelium, in a background of streaming mucous and blood. Salivary gland can be mistaken for an enlarged lymph node on physical exam. It is best to choose a node other than the submandibular node for aspiration, if there is multifocal lymphadenopathy, in order to avoid inadvertent submission of salivary tissue rather than lymph node.

Figure 2.70 shows a canine normal salivary gland biopsy. There are lobules of serous and mucous glands with a duct lined by cuboidal epithelium.

Salivary mucocele

Figure 2.71 shows a canine salivary gland mucocele FNA. Injury to a salivary gland or obstruction of a duct can result in release of mucin and saliva into adjacent stroma causing intense inflammation and formation of a firm submandibular mass. Typically there should be chronic inflammation, identified by the macrophages containing debris in this aspirate from a submandibular mass on a 5-year-old male Poodle. Often the macrophages contain phagocytosed erythrocytes, heme breakdown pigments, and sometimes hematoidin crystals. There should be clumps of mucin (arrow) in a background of erythrocytes and cellular debris.

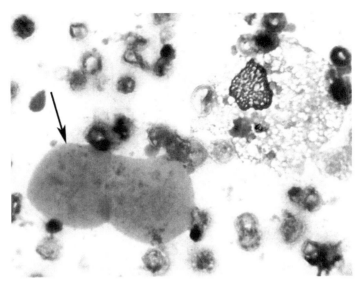

Figure 2.71 Canine salivary gland mucocele FNA. 50x.

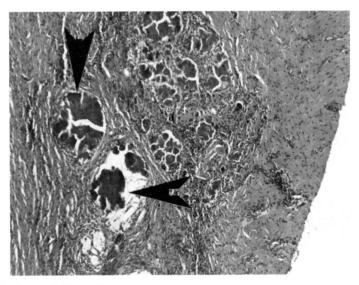

Figure 2.72 Canine salivary gland mucocele biopsy. 10x.

Figure 2.72 shows a biopsy of a canine salivary gland mucocele. Salivary fluid released into the stroma of this 3-year-old male Weimaraner results in tissue necrosis and an intense inflammatory infiltrate of macrophages, neutrophils, plasma cells, and small lymphocytes with areas of necrosis and fibrosis. The cause of this lesion is the lake of inspissated mucus and saliva (arrowhead) that has leaked from a damaged salivary gland.

Salivary gland carcinoma

Figure 2.73 shows a canine salivary gland carcinoma FNA. Aspiration of a salivary carcinoma causing a parotid area rapidly enlarging mass on an aged female mixed breed dog yielded large epithelioid cells with nuclear pleomorphism and basophilic cytoplasm in a background of abundant active macrophages and neutrophils. The cell at the upper right has two nuclei of different size, which is an indication of nuclear dysmaturation and a criterion of malignancy. At the bottom left center is nuclear debris and at the bottom right center is an active macrophage.

Figure 2.74 shows a biopsy of a canine salivary carcinoma. A mass associated with the right mandibular salivary gland of a neutered male German Shepherd mix of uncertain age was submitted. The salivary gland was mixed mucus and serous gland with extensive ischemic necrosis of one lobe and an adjacent salivary mucocele/sialocele surrounded by a scirrhous response. The poorly circumscribed infiltrative mass is comprised of islands of pleomorphic epithelial

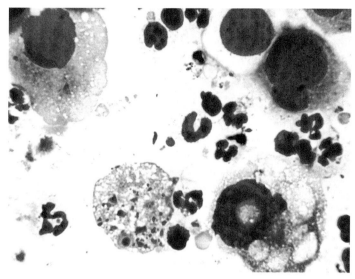

Figure 2.73 Canine salivary gland carcinoma FNA. 50x.

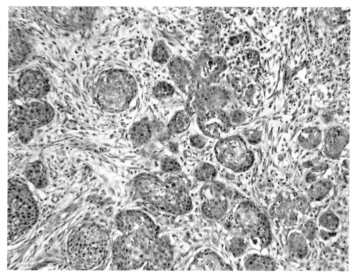

Figure 2.74 Canine salivary carcinoma biopsy. 10x.

cells that exhibit some central squamous differentiation and hints at keratinization. Some of the infiltrative glands have small lumina containing neutrophils. Most of the infiltrative cellular islands are solid. There is moderate variation in cell and nuclear size, and mitotic figures were occasionally seen in this cell population. Intralymphatic embolization was not recognized in the periphery available for examination. The inked margin on the section containing the mass was clean. Carcinomas are locally aggressive, they can recur even if completely resected, and they can metastasize via both blood vessels and lymphatics. Therefore, wide resection and careful follow-up are usually recommended.

Ventral neck masses

Ventral neck lesions are often due to thyroid disease, which is common in cats and sporadic in dogs. A thyroid mass in a cat is usually a result of hyperplasia or an adenoma. In a dog a thyroid mass is often a malignant thyroid tumor. Needle aspirate can reveal cells of presumptive thyroid origin that can help differentiate the mass from other mass lesions such as lymph nodes, vascular tumors, or stromal tumors. The complexity of nerve and vascular structures in this area can make biopsy a challenge so it is helpful to know if medical therapy could be the appropriate treatment.

Thyroid adenoma

Figure 2.75 shows an aspirate from a thyroid mass on a 9-year-old female Domestic Shorthair cat that yielded small clusters of cuboidal epithelium, sometimes appearing to form acini. On an initial presentation, with elevated serum T4 levels, a diagnosis of thyroid hyperplasia or adenoma would be appropriate, and medical therapy could be the preferred treatment.

Figure 2.76 shows a feline thyroid adenoma biopsy. A 14-year-old neutered male Domestic Shorthair cat was losing weight with good appetite and had an elevated T4. A left thyroidectomy was performed, as the left thyroid was considerably larger than the right. The thyroid was 2.5 × 1.0 × 0.8 cm with a discrete nodule. The specimen was bisected and totally submitted as two sections in one cassette. The adjacent normal thyroid tissue is actively secreting. The multilobular mass was discrete and circumscribed but not encapsulated. It is comprised of slightly enlarged thyroid follicular cells that line collapsed and dilated glands, usually in a single crowded layer. These glands contain pale eosinophilic secretion. The thyroid cells are mononuclear. They are slightly enlarged with slightly enlarged nuclei and a single nucleolus. No mitoses were seen after a moderate search. The mass appeared completely resected but partially peeled out. This thyroid mass is histologically benign. This functional tumor was responsible for the clinical signs. Occasionally thyroid adenomas are bilateral or multicentric, so periodic rechecks were advised.

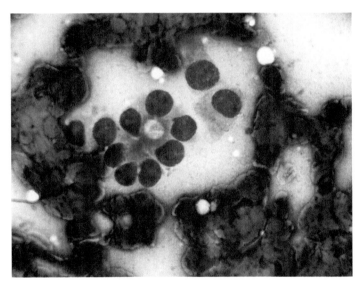

Figure 2.75 Feline thyroid adenoma FNA. 40x.

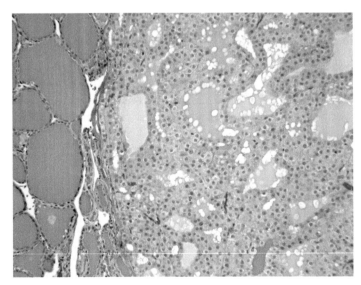

Figure 2.76 Feline thyroid adenoma biopsy. 10x.

Thyroid carcinoma

Figure 2.77 shows a canine thyroid carcinoma FNA. This aspirate is from a ventral cervical mass in a 12-year-old spayed female Spitz mix dog, that on initial presentation was 6 cm in length and firmly adhered to underlying structures. An aspirate revealed sheets of small epithelial cells with mild anisokaryosis, occasionally forming vague acinar structures.

Figure 2.78 shows a canine thyroid carcinoma biopsy. This is a sample taken postmortem from the mass described in Figure 2.77. The carotid artery and jugular vein were incorporated into the mass. There were areas of remaining identifiable thyroid acini, but most of the gland was effaced by sheets and nodules of small epithelial cells with mild anisokaryosis. There appeared to be vascular invasion. The invasive nature of the tumor was consistent with a carcinoma in spite of a fairly monomorphic cell population.

Parathyroid adenoma

Figure 2.79 shows a canine parathyroid adenoma FNA. Aspirate of thyroid area masses can reveal dense clusters of small epithelial cells with monomorphic nuclei and scant cytoplasm suggestive of basaloid or neuroendocrine epithelium. Formation of acini would not be expected because it would imply thyroid gland origin. Biopsy is necessary for definitive diagnosis.

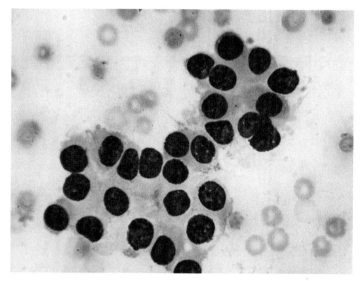

Figure 2.77 Canine thyroid carcinoma FNA. 50x.

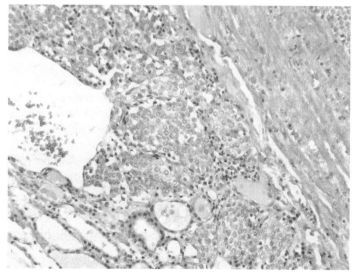

Figure 2.78 Canine thyroid carcinoma biopsy. 10x.

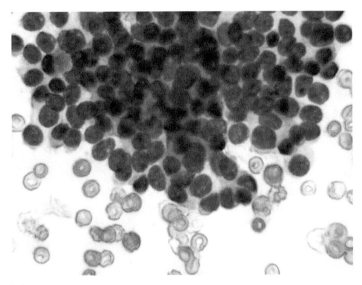

Figure 2.79 Canine parathyroid adenoma FNA. 50x.

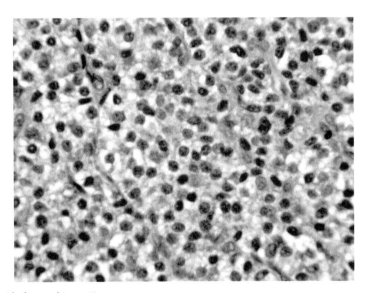

Figure 2.80 Canine parathyroid adenoma biopsy. 40x.

Figure 2.80 shows a biopsy of a canine parathyroid adenoma. A mass on the left side of the neck of a 12-year-old Beagle mix was submitted, bisected, totally submitted as two sections in one cassette, and processed for histopathology. This is an endocrine-type neoplasm consistent with a chief cell parathyroid adenoma. The mass was circumscribed with a narrow capsule. It is comprised of vague coalescing packets of fairly regular medium-sized polygonal cells with little variation in nuclear size, a modest amount of faintly vacuolated to finely granular eosinophilic cytoplasm, and distinct cell borders. The cells are mostly mononuclear. No mitoses were seen after a moderate search. No attached thyroid or lymph node tissue was recognized. The mass appeared partially peeled out. Parathyroid adenomas are usually found in elderly canines. Some affected patients have hypercalcemia. Nodular hyperplasia of the parathyroid glands results in a similar nodular mass or masses but is often bilateral and develops in some canines with chronic renal failure.

Additional reading

Bone tumors of the head

Barger AM. Musculoskeletal System. In Canine and Feline Cytology; A Color Atlas and Interpretation Guide. 3rd ed. Raskin and Meyer. 2016. Elsevier. St. Louis. 353–368.

Craig LE, Dittmer KE, Thompson KG. Bones and Joints. In Jubb, Kennedy, and Palmer's Pathology of Domestic Animals. Vol 1. 6th ed. M. Grant Maxie, Editor. Elsevier. St Louis. 2016. 16–163.

Ehrhart NP, Ryan SD, Fan TM. Tumors of the Skeletal System. In Small Animal Clinical Oncology, 5th ed. Withrow and MacEwen. 2013. Elsevier. St. Louis. 463–503.

Fielder SE. The Musculoskeletal System. In Cowell and Tyler's Diagnostic Cytology and Hematology of the Dog and Cat. 4th ed. Valenciano and Cowell. 2014. Elsevier. St. Louis. 216–221.

Mass lesions of the ear canal

Hauck ML. Tumors of the Skin and Subcutaneous tissues. In Tumors of the Skeletal System. In Small Animal Clinical Oncology, 5th ed. Withrow and MacEwen. 2013. Elsevier. St. Louis. 305–320.

Wallace KA, DeHeer H, Patel RT. The External Ear Canal. In Cowell and Tyler's Diagnostic Cytology and Hematology of the Dog and Cat. 4th ed. Valenciano and Cowell. 2014. Elsevier. St. Louis. 171–179.

Wilcox BP, Njaa BL. Special Senses. In Jubb, Kennedy, and Palmer's Pathology of Domestic Animals. Vol 1. 6th ed. M. Grant Maxie, Editor. Elsevier. St Louis. 2016. 407–508.

Ceruminous gland carcinoma

de Lorimier LP. Ceruminous Gland Adenocarcinoma, Ear. In Blackwell's Five-Minute Veterinary Consult: Canine and Feline. 5th ed. Tilley LP and Smith FWK, Jr. 2011. John Wiley & Sons, Inc. West Sussex, UK. 231.

Mass lesions of the external ear pinna

Hauck ML. Tumors of the Skin and Subcutaneous Tissues. In Small Animal Clinical Oncology, 5th ed. Withrow and MacEwen. 2013. Elsevier. St. Louis. 305–320.

Mauldin EA, Peters-Kennedy J. Integumentary System. In Jubb, Kennedy, and Palmer's Pathology of Domestic Animals. Vol 1. 6th ed. M. Grant Maxie, Editor. Elsevier. St Louis. 2016. 509–736.

Histiocytoma

Clifford CA. Histiocytoma. In Blackwell's Five-Minute Veterinary Consult: Canine and Feline. 5th ed. Tilley LP and Smith FWK, Jr. 2011. John Wiley & Sons, Inc. West Sussex, UK. 585.

Clifford CA, Skorupski KA, Moore PF. Histiocytic Diseases. In Small Animal Clinical Oncology, 5[th]ed. Withrow and MacEwen. 2013. Elsevier. St. Louis. 706–715.

Gross TL, Ihrke PJ, Walder EJ, and Affolter VK. Histiocytic Tumors. In Skin Diseases of the Dog and Cat; Clinical and Histopathologic Diagnosis. 2nd ed. 2005. Blackwell Publishing. Oxford. 837–852.

Squamous cell carcinoma

Gross TL, Ihrke PJ, Walder EJ, Affolter VK. Epidermal Tumors. In Skin Diseases of the Dog and Cat; Clinical and Histopathologic Diagnosis. 2nd ed. 2005. Blackwell Publishing. Oxford. 562–603.

Wypij JM. Squamous Cell Carcinoma, Ear. In Blackwell's Five-Minute Veterinary Consult: Canine and Feline. 5th ed. Tilley LP and Smith FWK, Jr. 2011. John Wiley & Sons, Inc. West Sussex, UK. 1184.

Mass lesions of the conjunctiva and nictitans

Gilger BC. Third Eyelid Protrusion. In Blackwell's Five-Minute Veterinary Consult: Canine and Feline. 5th ed. Tilley LP and Smith FWK, Jr. 2011. John Wiley & Sons, Inc. West Sussex, UK. 1223–1224.

Miller PE, Dubielzig RR. Ocular Tumors. In Small Animal Clinical Oncology, 5th ed. Withrow and MacEwen. 2013. Elsevier. St. Louis. 597–607.

Wilcox BP, Njaa BL. Special Senses. In Jubb, Kennedy, and Palmer's Pathology of Domestic Animals. Vol 1. 6th ed. M. Grant Maxie, Editor. Elsevier. St Louis. 2016. 407–508.

Young KM. Eyes and Associated Structures. In Cowell and Tyler's Diagnostic Cytology and Hematology of the Dog and Cat. 4th ed. Valenciano and Cowell. 2014. Elsevier. St. Louis. 150–170.

Eyelid masses

Miller PE, Dubielzig RR. Ocular Tumors. In Small Animal Clinical Oncology, 5th ed. Withrow and MacEwen. 2013. Elsevier. St. Louis. 597–607.

Meibomian gland adenoma
Wilcox BP, Njaa BL. Special Senses. In Jubb, Kennedy, and Palmer's Pathology of Domestic Animals. Vol 1. 6ᵗʰ ed. M. Grant Maxie, Editor. Elsevier. St Louis. 2016. 407–508.

Spindle cell tumor
Bell CM, Schwarz T, Dubielzig RR. Diagnostic Features of Feline Restrictive Orbital Myofibroblastic Sarcoma. Vet Path 2011; 48:742–750.

Lesions of the oral and nasal mucosal epithelium

Hauck ML. Tumors of the Skin and Subcutaneous Tissues. In Small Animal Clinical Oncology, 5th ed. Withrow and MacEwen. 2013. Elsevier. St. Louis. 305–320.
Liptak JM, Withrow SJ. Oral Tumors. In Small Animal Clinical Oncology, 5th ed. Withrow and MacEwen. 2013. Elsevier. St. Louis. 381–398.
Uzal FA, Plattner BL. Alimentary System. In Jubb, Kennedy and Palmer's Pathology of Domestic Animals. Vol 2. 6ᵗʰ ed. M. Grant Maxie, Editor. Elsevier. St Louis. 2016. 1–257.

Eosinophilic inflammation
Lymphoplasmacellular inflammation
Bellows J. Feline Oropharyngeal Inflammation. In Blackwell's Five-Minute Veterinary Consult: Canine and Feline. 5ᵗʰ ed. Tilley LP and Smith FWK, Jr. 2011. John Wiley & Sons, Inc. West Sussex, UK. 474.
Gross TL, Ihrke PJ, Walder EJ, Affolter VK. Ulcerative and Crusting Diseases of the Epidermis. In Skin Diseases of the Dog and Cat; Clinical and Histopathologic Diagnosis. 2ⁿᵈ ed. 2005. Blackwell Publishing. Oxford. 116–135.
Peak RM. Oral Ulceration. In Blackwell's Five-Minute Veterinary Consult: Canine and Feline. 5ᵗʰ ed. Tilley LP and Smith FWK, Jr. 2011. John Wiley & Sons, Inc. West Sussex, UK. 911–912.
Werner AH. Eosinophilic Granuloma Complex. In Blackwell's Five-Minute Veterinary Consult: Canine and Feline. 5ᵗʰ ed. Tilley LP and Smith FWK, Jr. 2011. John Wiley & Sons, Inc. West Sussex, UK. 420–421.

Acanthomatous epulis
Morrison WB. Ameloblastoma. In Blackwell's Five-Minute Veterinary Consult: Canine and Feline. 5ᵗʰ ed. Tilley LP and Smith FWK, Jr. 2011. John Wiley & Sons, Inc. West Sussex, UK. 61.

Viral papilloma
Gross TL, Ihrke PJ, Walder EJ, Affolter VK. Epidermal Tumors. In Skin Diseases of the Dog and Cat; Clinical and Histopathologic Diagnosis. 2ⁿᵈ ed. 2005. Blackwell Publishing. Oxford. 562–603.

Squamous cell carcinoma
Withrow SJ. Cancer of the Nasal Planum. In Small Animal Clinical Oncology, 5th ed. Withrow and MacEwen. 2013. Elsevier. St. Louis. 432–435.
Wypij JM. Squamous Cell Carcinoma, Gingiva. In Blackwell's Five-Minute Veterinary Consult: Canine and Feline. 5ᵗʰ ed. Tilley LP and Smith FWK, Jr. 2011. John Wiley & Sons, Inc. West Sussex, UK. 1185.

Melanoma
Bergman PJ, Kent MS, Farese JP. Melanoma. In Small Animal Clinical Oncology, 5th ed. Withrow and MacEwen. 2013. Elsevier. St. Louis. 321–334.
de Lorimier LP. Melanocytic Tumors, Oral. In Blackwell's Five-Minute Veterinary Consult: Canine and Feline. 5ᵗʰ ed. Tilley LP and Smith FWK, Jr. 2011. John Wiley & Sons, Inc. West Sussex, UK. 807.

Nasal cavity tumors

Arndt TP. Nasal Exudates and Masses. In Cowell and Tyler's Diagnostic Cytology and Hematology of the Dog and Cat. 4ᵗʰ ed. Valenciano and Cowell. 2014. Elsevier. St. Louis. 131–138.
Burkhard MJ. Respiratory Tract. In Canine and Feline Cytology; A Color Atlas and Interpretation Guide. 3ʳᵈ ed. Raskin and Meyer. 2016. Elsevier. St. Louis. 138–190.
Caswell JL, Williams KJ. Respiratory System. In Jubb, Kennedy and Palmer's Pathology of Domestic Animals. Vol 2. 6ᵗʰ ed. M. Grant Maxie, Editor. Elsevier. St Louis. 2016. 465–591.
Turek MM, Lana SE. Nasosinal Tumors. In Small Animal Clinical Oncology, 5th ed. Withrow and MacEwen. 2013. Elsevier. St. Louis. 435–451.

Adenocarcinoma

De Lorimier LP. Adenocarcinoma, Nasal. In Blackwell's Five-Minute Veterinary Consult: Canine and Feline. 5th ed. Tilley LP and Smith FWK, Jr. 2011. John Wiley & Sons, Inc. West Sussex, UK. 26.

Chondrosarcoma

Bailey DB. Chondrosarcoma, Nasal and Paranasal Sinus. In Blackwell's Five-Minute Veterinary Consult: Canine and Feline. 5th ed. Tilley LP and Smith FWK, Jr. 2011. John Wiley & Sons, Inc. West Sussex, UK. 252.

Mass lesions of the canine and feline muzzle skin

Fisher DJ. Cutaneous and Subcutaneous Lesions. In Cowell and Tyler's Diagnostic Cytology and Hematology of the Dog and Cat. 4th ed. Valenciano and Cowell. 2014. Elsevier. St. Louis. 80–109.

Hauck ML. Tumors of the Skin and Subcutaneous Tissues. In Small Animal Clinical Oncology, 5th ed. Withrow and MacEwen. 2013. Elsevier. St. Louis. 305–320.

Mauldin EA, Peters-Kennedy J. Integumentary System. In Jubb, Kennedy and Palmer's Pathology of Domestic Animals. Vol 1. 6th ed. M. Grant Maxie, Editor. Elsevier. St Louis. 2016. 509–736.

Raskin RE. Skin and Subcutaneous Tissues. In Canine and Feline Cytology; A Color Atlas and Interpretation Guide. 3rd ed. Raskin and Meyer. 2016. Elsevier. St. Louis. 34–90.

Sebaceous gland nodular hyperplasia
Sebaceous gland adenoma
Sebaceous epithelioma

Gross TL, Ihrke PJ, Walder EJ, Affolter VK. Sebaceous Tumors. In Skin Diseases of the Dog and Cat; Clinical and Histopathologic Diagnosis. 2nd ed. 2005. Blackwell Publishing. Oxford. 641–664.

Trichoblastoma (Basal cell tumor)

Gross TL, Ihrke PJ, Walder EJ, Affolter VK. Epidermal Tumors. In Skin Diseases of the Dog and Cat; Clinical and Histopathologic Diagnosis. 2nd ed. 2005. Blackwell Publishing. Oxford. 562–603.

Mast cell tumor

Gross TL, Ihrke PJ, Walder EJ, Affolter VK. Mast Cell Tumors. In Skin Diseases of the Dog and Cat; Clinical and Histopathologic Diagnosis. 2nd ed. 2005. Blackwell Publishing. Oxford. 853–865.

London CA, Thamm DH. Mast Cell Tumors. In Small Animal Clinical Oncology, 5th ed. Withrow and MacEwen. 2013. Elsevier. St. Louis. 335–355.

Plasma cell tumor

Gross TL, Ihrke PJ, Walder EJ, Affolter VK. Lymphocytic Tumors. In Skin Diseases of the Dog and Cat; Clinical and Histopathologic Diagnosis. 2nd ed. 2005. Blackwell Publishing. Oxford. 866–893.

Vail DM. Myeloma-Related Disorders. In Small Animal Clinical Oncology, 5th ed. Withrow and MacEwen. 2013. Elsevier. St. Louis. 665–678.

Mass lesions of the submandibular region

Reactive lymph node
Malignant lymphoma

Messick JB. The Lymph Nodes. In Cowell and Tyler's Diagnostic Cytology and Hematology of the Dog and Cat. 4th ed. Valenciano and Cowell. 2014. Elsevier. St. Louis. 180–194.

Raskin RE. Hemolymphatic System. In Canine and Feline Cytology; A Color Atlas and Interpretation Guide. 3rd ed. Raskin and Meyer. 2016. Elsevier. St. Louis. 91–137.

Vail DM, Pinkerton ME, Young KE. Canine Lymphoma and Lymphoid Leukemias. In Small Animal Clinical Oncology, 5th ed. Withrow and MacEwen. 2013. Elsevier. St. Louis. 608–638.

Valli VEO, Kiupel M, Bienzle D. Hematopoietic System. In Jubb, Kennedy and Palmer's Pathology of Domestic Animals. Vol 3. 6th ed. M. Grant Maxie, Editor. Elsevier. St Louis. 2016. 102–268.

Normal salivary gland
Salivary mucocele
Allison RW. Subcutaneous Glandular Tissue: Mammary, Salivary, Thyroid and Parathyroid. In Cowell and Tyler's Diagnostic Cytology and Hematology of the Dog and Cat. 4th ed. Valenciano and Cowell. 2014. Elsevier. St. Louis. 110–130.
Lauer SK. Salivary Mucocele. In Blackwell's Five-Minute Veterinary Consult: Canine and Feline. 5th ed. Tilley LP and Smith FWK, Jr. 2011. John Wiley & Sons, Inc. West Sussex, UK. 1124–1125.

Salivary gland carcinoma
Mutsaers AJ. Adenocarcinoma, Salivary Gland. In Blackwell's Five-Minute Veterinary Consult: Canine and Feline. 5th ed. Tilley LP and Smith FWK, Jr. 2011. John Wiley & Sons, Inc. West Sussex, UK. 30.
Withrow SJ. Salivary Gland Cancer. In Small Animal Clinical Oncology, 5th ed. Withrow and MacEwen. 2013. Elsevier. St. Louis. 398–399.

Ventral neck masses

Allison RW. Subcutaneous Glandular Tissue: Mammary, Salivary, Thyroid and Parathyroid. In Cowell and Tyler's Diagnostic Cytology and Hematology of the Dog and Cat. 4th ed. Valenciano and Cowell. 2014. Elsevier. St. Louis. 110–130.
Choi US, Arndt T. Endocrine/Neuroendocrine System. In Canine and Feline Cytology; A Color Atlas and Interpretation Guide. 3rd ed. Raskin and Meyer. 2016. Elsevier. St. Louis. 430–452.
Lunn KF, Page RL. Tumors of the Endocrine System. In Small Animal Clinical Oncology, 5th ed. Withrow and MacEwen. 2013. Elsevier. St. Louis. 504–531.
Rosol, TJ, Grone A. Endocrine Glands. In Jubb, Kennedy and Palmer's Pathology of Domestic Animals. Vol 3. 6th ed. M. Grant Maxie, Editor. Elsevier. St Louis. 2016. 269–357.

Thyroid carcinoma
Newman RG. Adenocarcinoma, Thyroid-Dogs. In Blackwell's Five-Minute Veterinary Consult: Canine and Feline. 5th ed. Tilley LP and Smith FWK, Jr. 2011. John Wiley & Sons, Inc. West Sussex, UK. 33–34.

3 Selected Lesions of the Limbs, Paws, and Digits

Inflammatory, hyperplastic, and neoplastic lesions of the limbs and feet can present as obvious lameness or may be discovered as a result of subtle clinical signs such as drops of blood on the bedding or furniture. A thick hair coat can mask a lesion until these symptoms result in the discovery of an enlarging mass.

Bone lesions

Bone is a metabolically active tissue that responds to injury of any kind with a proliferative attempt at repair. Even neoplastic bone can have associated reactive bone as the adjacent normal bone attempts to repair damage due to instability or necrosis. This can complicate the diagnostic process, and it is often necessary to utilize all tools available, including history, radiographs, FNA, and biopsy to obtain a definitive diagnosis and prognosis.

Periosteal hyperplasia
Figure 3.1 shows a radiograph of periosteal hyperplasia. Periosteal hyperplasia can be seen with healing fractures and thoracic masses. Radiology reveals an organized mineralized lacy pattern at the bone margins (arrow) with minimal evidence of destruction or disorganized proliferation of bone.

Figure 3.2 shows a periosteal hyperplasia FNA. Aspiration in the area of proliferative bone indicated by the arrow in Figure 3.1 may yield abundant metachromatic bone matrix encompassing nucleated cells with small, single nuclei and mild anisokaryosis. These cells appear to be chondroblasts or osteoblasts. They do not exhibit features of malignancy, but biopsy would be necessary to evaluate the architecture.

Figure 3.3 shows a periosteal hyperplasia biopsy. Biopsy in the area indicated by the arrow on Figure 3.1 reveals a proliferation of well-differentiated trabecular bone emerging from the cortical bone and pushing against the soft tissue of the limb. FNA of this type of periosteal hyperplasia or reactive bone can be poorly cellular or may reveal metachromatic osteoid and small epithelioid osteoblasts and/or chondroblasts.

Osteosarcoma
Figure 3.4 shows a radiograph of an osteosarcoma in the distal radius of a dog revealing areas of bone proliferation and lysis and breach of the cortical bone. Biopsy should be taken at the arrow site.

Figure 3.5 shows a canine osteosarcoma FNA. Aspirate of a lytic bone lesion at the arrow site can yield varying combinations of blood, spindle cells, multinucleate cells compatible with osteoclasts, and large epithelioid cells compatible with osteoblasts or chondroblasts. This high-density, mixed osteoprogenitor population, when present with areas of eosinophilic matrix, is suggestive of bone proliferation. When these cells are typical in appearance it is difficult to make a diagnosis of neoplasia using cytology alone. Clinical history is important for accurate interpretation of bone lesions. A dense population of osteoprogenitor cells with large variations in nuclear size (moderate to marked anisokaryosis) suggests a neoplastic process if there is not another clinically apparent reason for active bone production, such as a fracture or infectious agent.

Figure 3.6 shows a biopsy of a canine humeral osteosarcoma. A 9-year-old spayed female Labrador Retriever mix was presented with non-weight-bearing lameness, atrophy of the scapulohumeral muscles, and pain in the left forelimb.

Atlas for the Diagnosis of Tumors in the Dog and Cat, First Edition. Anita R. Kiehl and Maron Brown Calderwood Mays.
© 2016 John Wiley & Sons, Inc. Published 2016 by John Wiley & Sons, Inc.

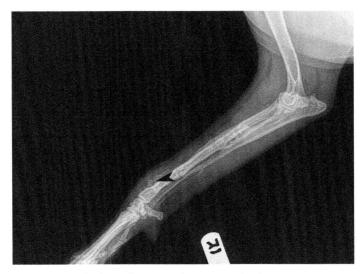

Figure 3.1 Radiograph of periosteal hyperplasia. (Radiograph courtesy of Dr. Laura Hokett.)

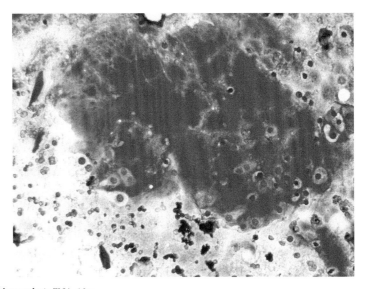

Figure 3.2 Canine periosteal hyperplasia FNA. 10x.

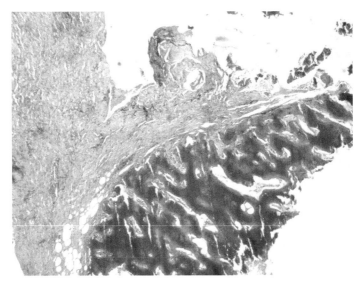

Figure 3.3 Periosteal hyperplasia biopsy. 2.5x.

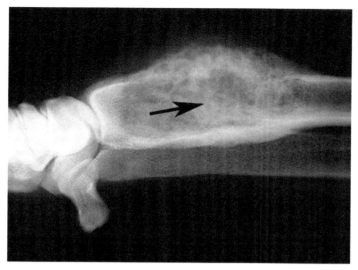

Figure 3.4 Radiograph of canine osteosarcoma. (Radiograph courtesy of Dr. Rowan Milner.)

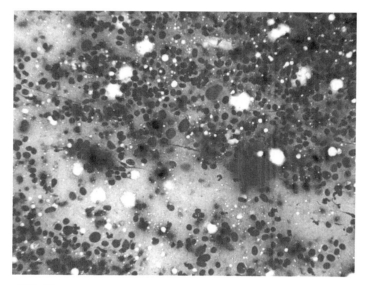

Figure 3.5 Canine osteosarcoma FNA. 10x.

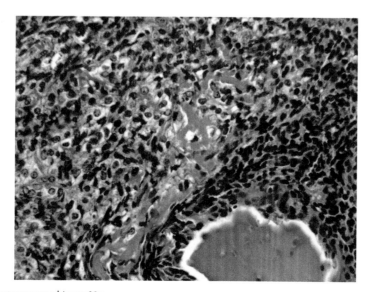

Figure 3.6 Canine humeral osteosarcoma biopsy. 20x.

Radiographs revealed proliferative and lytic cortical bone in the proximal caudal left humeral metaphysis. The clinical diagnosis was osteosarcoma with a differential diagnosis of osteomyelitis, and the owner elected amputation. Two punch biopsies of the affected area in the humerus were submitted. Only a portion of the intertrabecular spaces was involved in each specimen. In these areas the intertrabecular spaces are filled by sheets of discrete medium to fairly large polygonal cells that appeared osteoblastic. There is some variation in cell nuclear size, and the cells are mostly mononuclear. Mitotic figures were found in this cell population. These cells multifocally deposit intensely eosinophilic osteoid. There is also a fragment of non-neoplastic bone in the photomicrograph. There was very little stroma in the involved cellular intertrabecular areas. The histology is consistent with osteoblastic osteosarcoma. These tumors are locally aggressive, many of them metastasize early to the lungs, and they can also metastasize to regional lymph nodes. They occasionally recur at the amputation site.

Subungual tumors

Melanoma

Figure 3.7 shows a canine melanoma FNA. Aspirate of a melanoma can yield spindloid poorly granulated melanocytes, or plump epithelioid and densely granulated melanocytes, depending on the area of aspiration. This tumor type is very heterogeneous and can exhibit wide variation in cell appearance. Melanocytic tumors of the skin, and in this instance a subungual mass, may yield slender spindle cells with occasional faintly granular cytoplasm. It may be necessary to look for any melanin granules at the highest power, on oil, for diagnosis of poorly melanotic tumors.

Figure 3.8 shows an excisional biopsy of a subungual mass from the left rear third digit of a 12-year-old well cared for Dachshund, the same mass aspirated in Figure 3.7. Grossly the mass had the appearance of a tick, but aspiration had revealed scattered melanocytes, and removal proved it to be a poorly melanotic spindloid melanoma with a mitotic rate of 0–1/HPF and a mitotic index of less than 1/10 HPF. Rare junctional nesting was seen, confirming the diagnosis of melanoma. Subungual melanomas are often very aggressive, but this tumor was considered to be well differentiated and likely non-aggressive based on the low mitotic rate and lack of invasion into underlying bone. Excision was complete with wide margins and there was no evidence of further disease at 3 years. This case demonstrates how FNA can be a useful clue that a lesion that appears benign on gross exam has a more aggressive potential than assumed, allowing complete removal of this melanoma at an early stage with no recurrence.

Figure 3.9 shows a canine nail bed melanoma FNA. Aspiration of a subungual mass on an adult spayed female mixed breed dog revealed clusters of spindloid to epithelioid cells with moderate anisokaryosis and moderate to dense cytoplasmic melanin. Biopsy was recommended to determine the mitotic index and look for invasion into underlying bone.

Figure 3.10 shows a canine subungual malignant melanoma biopsy. An 8-year-old spayed female Labrador Retriever developed a destructive lesion in the third phalanx of the left front fifth digit, accompanied by a proliferative reaction on

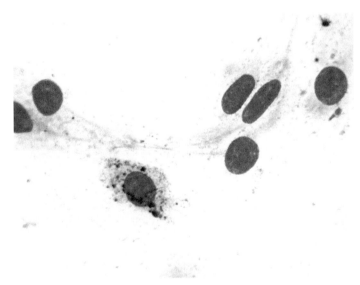

Figure 3.7 Canine melanoma FNA. 40x.

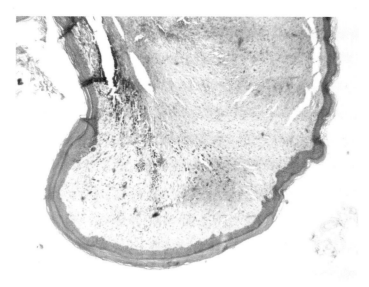

Figure 3.8 Canine subungual melanoma biopsy. 2.5x.

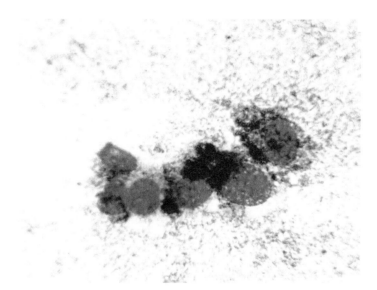

Figure 3.9 Canine nail bed melanoma FNA. 40x.

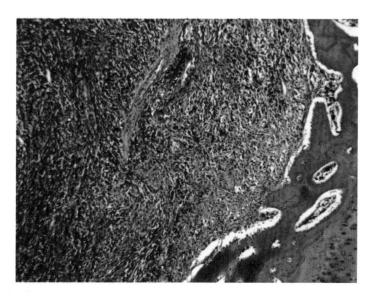

Figure 3.10 Canine subungual malignant melanoma biopsy. 20x.

the lateral second phalanx. The digit was amputated at the metacarpal-phalangeal joint. The submitted amputated digit had a protruding normal P1, a split dysplastic claw, and an ulcerated mass displacing the claw and involving the medial surface of the distal digit. The claw and P1 were removed, and the distal digit was sawed in half sagittally, revealing a multilobular black mass that effaced the nail bed and P3, with encroachment on distal P2. This neoplasm had been completely resected with a proximal soft tissue margin of 0.8 cm. One trimmed representative sagittal section through the mass was examined histologically. The surface of the large mass was extensively ulcerated. It is a multilobular neoplasm comprised of pleomorphic medium to large polygonal and plump spindloid cells, many of which are heavily pigmented. There is moderate variation in cell and nuclear size, and some cells have more than one nucleus. Mitoses were seen at a rate of 0–3/HPF, depending on area. The nail bed was unrecognizable, and most of P3 had been destroyed. These tumors are locally aggressive. They can recur at a later date at the amputation site. Metastasis to regional lymph nodes and then to the lungs and other sites can occur even if the original resection was complete and timely.

Squamous cell carcinoma

Figure 3.11 shows a canine squamous cell carcinoma FNA. Aspirate of a left front third digit subungual mass lesion on an adult male mixed breed dog yielded epithelial cells of varying size with abundant basophilic to clear cytoplasm, moderate to marked anisokaryosis, and nuclear/cytoplasmic dysmaturation (the nucleus should become pyknotic as the cytoplasm clears, rendering the cell metabolically inactive as it moves to the surface of the epidermis), suggesting a population of cells that are not maturing normally and may be experiencing uncontrolled growth. Several squamous cells have a large nucleus in clear cytoplasm, a sign of significant dysmaturation and a hallmark of this type of carcinoma. There are often many neutrophils in a background of cellular debris, as this lesion lacks the normal protective keratin layer of normal skin, and there is usually a fairly dense interface inflammatory infiltrate.

Figure 3.12 shows a canine subungual squamous cell carcinoma biopsy. An amputated right hind third digit with missing claw and a 1.7-cm-diameter ulcer where the claw should be located was submitted from a 10-year-old neutered male Giant Schnauzer. The specimen was sawed in half longitudinally, revealing an ill-defined white/tan/brown nail bed mass that had been completely resected with a narrowest proximal margin of 0.7 cm. A representative section of the mass was examined histologically. Suppurative granulation tissue is proliferating in the distal ulcer bed. The mass has a moderately cellular fibrovascular stroma that is multifocally inflamed. It is comprised of infiltrative nodules and anastomosing trabeculae of pleomorphic neoplastic squamous epithelium with central keratinization, dyskeratosis, and the formation of keratin pearls. Margins on the section were clean. This mass is a subungual squamous cell carcinoma. These tumors are locally aggressive, so amputation is the treatment of choice. Even with timely complete resection, metastasis to regional lymph nodes and the lungs occasionally occurs. There is an increased incidence in this breed.

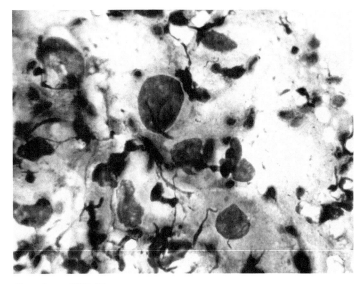

Figure 3.11 Canine squamous cell carcinoma FNA. 50x.

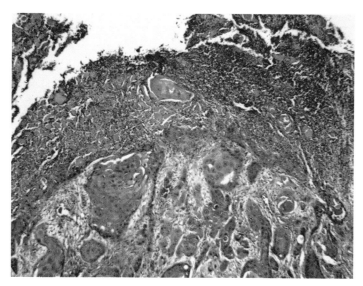

Figure 3.12 Canine subungual squamous cell carcinoma biopsy. 4x.

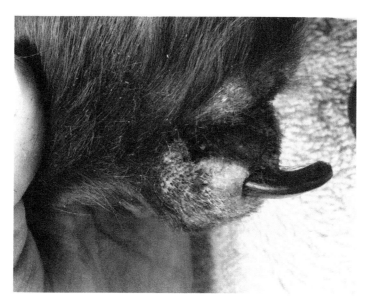

Figure 3.13 Clinical photograph of shaved digital mass.

Digital skin and nail bed lesions

Figure 3.13 is a clinical photograph of a shaved digital mass. This mass on the toe of a dog was not evident until the digit was shaved. The presenting complaint was a painful paw.

Calcinosis circumscripta

Figure 3.14 shows a calcinosis circumscripta FNA. This lesion may present as multiple firm masses on the distal extremities. A 3-year-old neutered male German Shepherd Dog presented with multiple small masses on the distal lateral left front paw. Aspiration yielded a few active macrophages in a background of amorphous refractile debris when examined under 50x with oil.

Figure 3.15 shows a calcinosis circumscripta biopsy. Biopsy of a mass on the hock of a young male Great Dane revealed dense foci of mineralized debris surrounded by a wall of fibrosis occasionally containing macrophages and neutrophils typical of calcinosis circumscripta. This lesion can present as single to multiple firm, multinodular masses on extremities, pressure points, and sometimes ear tips. It is more common in large breed dogs. It may be a result of traumatic injury and dystrophic calcification. It is benign and complete excision should be curative.

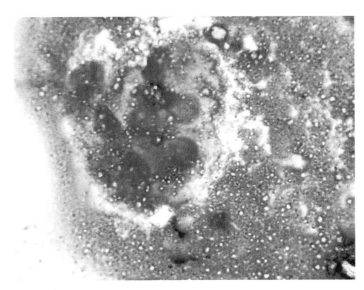

Figure 3.14 Calcinosis circumscripta FNA. 50x.

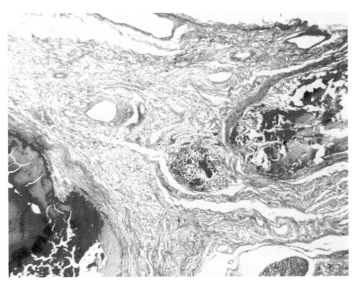

Figure 3.15 Calcinosis circumscripta biopsy. 2.5x.

Plasmacellular pododermatitis

Figure 3.16 shows a plasmacellular pododermatitis FNA. An adult spayed female Domestic Shorthair cat presented with multiple swollen pink paw pads. Aspirate of plasmacellular pododermatitis often yields mostly plasma cells with a few small lymphocytes, occasional neutrophils, and rarely eosinophils. Globulin-laden plasma cells, Mott cells (arrow), can be seen. This mixed population suggests an allergic response to antigenic stimulation. If eosinophils predominate suspect eosinophilic granuloma instead.

Figure 3.17 shows a biopsy of a feline plasmacellular pododermatitis. A 10-year-old spayed female Domestic Shorthair cat presented with ulcerated paw pads of multiple feet, which tended to wax and wane. Biopsy revealed multifocal variable erosion and ulceration of the pad epidermis with dense dermal infiltrates of plasma cells with a few lymphocytes and only rare eosinophils.

Papilloma

A common superficial epithelial tumor is papilloma, which is caused by a group of infectious viruses. Papillomas are more common in young dogs and immunocompromised animals. They may spontaneously regress or become multiple. When a papilloma arises in the confined space of the nail bed, especially in the subungual region, it may cause pressure necrosis of P3, inflammation, pain, and lameness. Other, more aggressive tumors, occur frequently in the

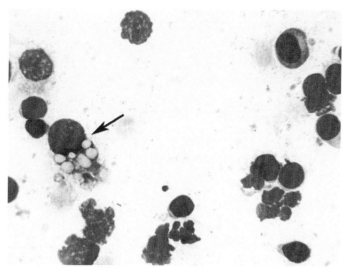

Figure 3.16 Plasmacellular pododermatitis FNA. 40x.

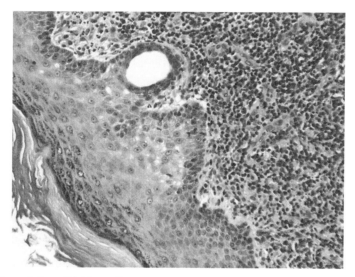

Figure 3.17 Feline plasmacellular pododermatitis biopsy. 10x.

subungual region, and digital amputation may be the most appropriate course in order to obtain a representative biopsy for accurate prognosis.

Figure 3.18 shows a canine papilloma cytology. FNA, scrapes, or impressions of papillomas will yield mostly mature squamous epithelium with occasional dyskeratosis and variably pleomorphic nuclei resulting from viral-induced nuclear activity, as seen in this scrape from a toe mass on an 8-year-old spayed female Labrador Retriever. There can be many neutrophils if the lesion is traumatized.

Figure 3.19 shows a biopsy of a canine inverted viral papilloma. A 7-year-old spayed female Doberman Pinscher suddenly developed a raised 11-mm-diameter mass on the dorsal surface of the left hind second digit. The mass was raised with a slightly narrower base. It had multiple cup-shaped epithelial invaginations. In the photomicrograph is one cup-shaped invagination of thick stratified squamous epithelium with inward keratinization, which is partly parakeratotic. In and near the granular layer in the area of inward keratinization there are swollen epithelial cells called koilocytes, with increased pale amphophilic cytoplasm (viral cytopathic effects.) Ghosts of these swollen cells are numerous in the keratin plug within the central invagination. Margins on the sections were clean. Canine viral papillomas are frequently multiple and sometimes numerous. The inverted variety is seen most often on canine feet. The owner was notified that young canines exposed to this patient may be susceptible to the papillomavirus infection.

Figure 3.20 shows a canine subungual inverted papilloma biopsy. An 8-year-old spayed female Labrador dog presented for lameness of the left forelimb. The medial digit was swollen and painful, and biopsy revealed that an

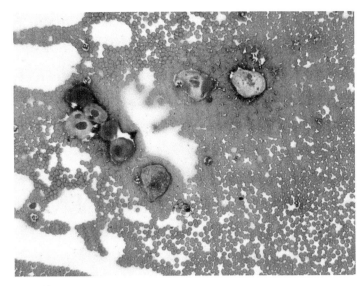

Figure 3.18 Canine papilloma scrape. 10x.

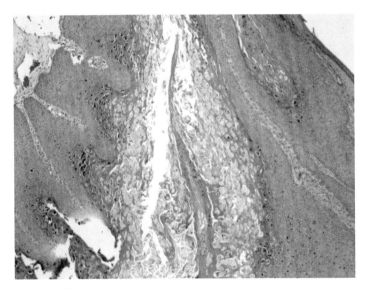

Figure 3.19 Canine inverted viral papilloma biopsy. 4x.

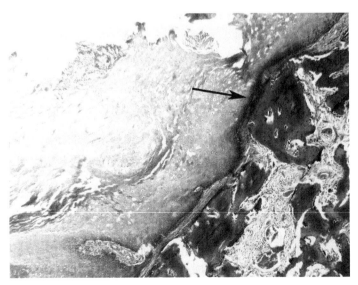

Figure 3.20 Canine subungual inverted papilloma biopsy. 2.5x.

inverted papilloma had arisen in the nail bed and created pressure on the bone of the third phalanx (arrow), resulting in distortion of the distal phalange and causing osteoarthritis of the joint, swelling, and pain. Amputation of the digit relieved the pain, and the lameness resolved.

Fibroadnexal hyperplasia

The adnexal structures of the digital skin can form cysts or cystic tumors that fill with keratin or secretory material. The digits are frequently exposed to traumatic injury because there is little subcutaneous fat. This can result in rupture of the cystic lesion with cellulitis due to release of cyst contents into the stroma. Complete excision while the lesion is still small is warranted. FNA can provide a tentative diagnosis of the cause of the lesion, which can be helpful to estimate the size of the margins necessary for cure.

Figure 3.21 shows a fibroadnexal hamartoma FNA. This lesion can present as a firm mass in the skin and may yield a few scattered spindle cells from the fibrous tissue around the lesion, keratin from the cystic center, and rare sebaceous, ductular, or squamous epithelial cells from the adnexal structures. Aspirate of a mass on the dorsal carpus of an adult spayed female Doberman Pinscher, which was clinically diagnosed as a "lick granuloma," revealed mostly scattered slender spindle cells and a few small epithelioid in scant blood.

Figure 3.22 shows a canine fibroadnexal hamartoma biopsy. A 10-year-old male Beagle had an ulcerated mass on the dorsal distal aspect of left carpus. The circumscribed fibrous nodule contains enlarged pilosebaceous units rendered

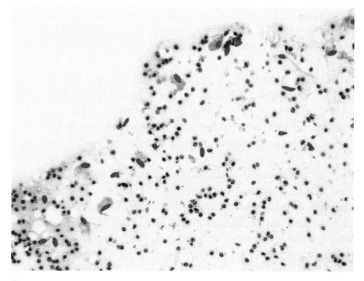

Figure 3.21 Canine fibroadnexal hamartoma FNA. 10x.

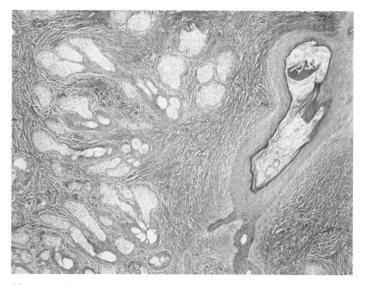

Figure 3.22 Canine fibroadnexal hamartoma biopsy. 4x.

somewhat dysplastic by the fibrosis. Follicular rupture had incited two foreign body responses containing keratin flakes and at least one hair shaft fragment. One of these inflammatory foci extended into the deep margin of the specimen. The fibrous nodule was circumscribed and appeared completely resected. This firm skin mass is sometimes called a fibroadnexal hamartoma. Inflammation is a common complication. The term hamartoma implies a congenital lesion, which seems unlikely in this case. These benign fibrous nodules can also be acquired secondary to an injury, and they may be multiple. They tend to develop in areas of chronic irritation or repeated trauma, possibly self-trauma in this location. Complete resection is usually curative for individual such nodules if there is not ongoing self-mutilation by chewing (lick granuloma).

Stromal tumors of the limb

Soft tissue sarcomas can originate from fibroblasts, nerves, adipocytes, joint capsule, or any structural component of the limb. Their behavior ranges from benign to aggressive. FNA can sometimes give an estimated prognosis of the behavior of the tumor if aspirated cells demonstrate criteria of malignancy. Early excision is suggested because there is little tissue available for surgical margins if the biopsy shows the tumor to be aggressive and high grade or if it is incompletely excised. Referral to a surgical specialist could be offered when the mass is in an area that may be difficult to completely remove.

Figure 3.23 is a clinical photograph of a canine hock with a subcutaneous mass. This soft tissue mass revealed spindle cells on aspiration. Spindle cell tumors at this site are often difficult to remove completely because they grow around tendon sheaths and nerves. Incomplete excision without further intervention usually results in progressively more aggressive regrowth with limb amputation as the final result.

Canine low-grade spindle cell tumor

Figure 3.24 shows a canine spindle cell tumor FNA. Aspirate of a mass on the hock of an adult neutered male Boxer mix dog revealed a variably dense population of slender spindle cells, some in small clusters, in scant blood. Low-grade canine spindle cell tumors of various types result in a cytologic picture of benign appearing slender spindle cells, but the cells may shed in small clumps, a behavior that is not typical of normal tissue. Anisokaryosis is often mild but may be moderate.

Figure 3.25 shows a canine fibroma biopsy. A small firm mass from a lateral hind leg of a 4-year-old neutered male Pit Bull Terrier was submitted. This fibrous mass was fairly well circumscribed but not encapsulated. It is comprised of thick intersecting collagen bundles rather sparsely populated by small to medium spindle cells that appear fibroblastic. There is mild variation in cell and nuclear size. The cytoplasm blends into the dense collagenous stroma. Most cells are mononuclear. One mitotic figure was seen after a moderate search. Margins were clean but narrow. These benign tumors may be dermal or subcutaneous. They are occasionally multiple. Complete resection should be curative.

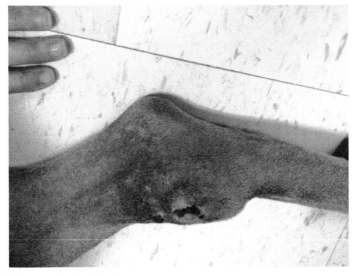

Figure 3.23 Clinical photograph of a canine hock with a subcutaneous mass.

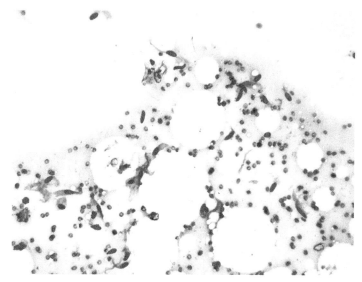

Figure 3.24 Canine spindle cell tumor FNA. 10x.

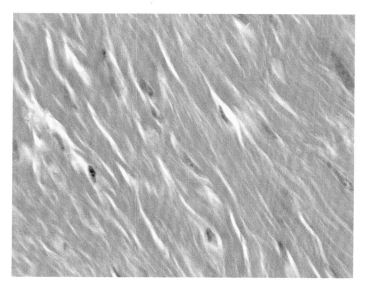

Figure 3.25 Canine fibroma biopsy. 40x.

Figure 3.26 shows a canine grade 1 neurofibrosarcoma biopsy. A mass was present for 4 months on the lateral right hock of a 12-year-old spayed female Boxer. This tissue is a multilobular mass of neoplastic polygonal and plump spindle cells. The cells are organized in interlacing bundles, swirls, and herringbone patterns. The area pictured is very cellular with little stroma. In other areas the cells were more loosely arranged with moderate amounts of collagen. The cells have oval to elongated nuclei with one or two nucleoli. Mitoses were seen in low numbers, but multinucleated cells were sometimes noted. Cytoplasm is generally eosinophilic and streaming with indistinct cell borders. The mass extended multifocally into the margins, appearing peeled out. Scores: Differentiation, suspect nerve sheath origin = 2; mitoses, 2/10 HPF = 1; necrosis, none = 1. Total = 4. Grade 1. The spindle cell tumors are difficult to differentiate by light microscopy. The most common differentials include fibrosarcoma, canine hemangiopericytoma, and tumors of nerve or nerve sheath origin (neurofibroma, neurofibrosarcoma, schwannoma.) Nerve sheath origin was suspected in this case because of cytologic features and proliferative pattern. Neurofibrosarcomas are usually solitary, occasionally multinodular along a nerve branch, and rarely multicentric. All of these tumors are slow to metastasize but are famous for local recurrence. Therefore, radical resection and careful follow-up are usually recommended.

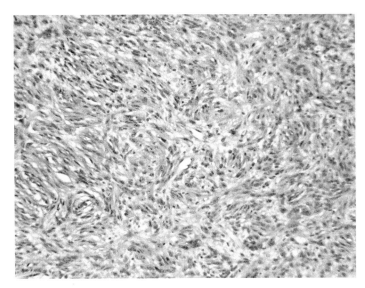

Figure 3.26 Canine grade 1 neurofibrosarcoma biopsy. 10x.

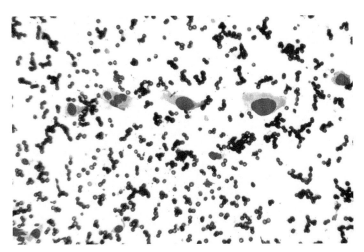

Figure 3.27 Feline spindle cell tumor FNA. 10x.

Feline spindle cell tumor

Figure 3.27 shows a feline spindle cell tumor FNA. FNA of canine and feline high-grade spindle cell tumors can yield spindle cell populations with moderate to marked anisokaryosis, multiple nuclei, prominent nucleoli, and variably basophilic cytoplasm. This aspirate of a mass from the paw of an adult neutered male Domestic Shorthair cat revealed spindle cells with moderate anisokaryosis and lightly basophilic spindloid cytoplasm with occasional multinucleate cells in a background of blood with minimal inflammation. Sometimes only rare cells are seen, and the slide should be searched for any multinucleate cells or cells with moderate anisokaryosis because the presence of even one cell with this appearance is a warning that biopsy should be performed in a timely fashion. This tumor type spreads quickly along fascial planes and must be completely removed while as small as possible. Advanced imaging techniques can be helpful to determine the true extent of the tumor. Limb amputation is often necessary if the tumor has become too large for local removal.

Figure 3.28 shows a biopsy of a feline fibrosarcoma. This mass is from the right front leg of a 10-year-old spayed female Domestic Medium Hair cat. The mass was a multilobular spindle cell neoplasm. In viable areas the cells are organized in vague broad interlacing bundles. In the pictured areas the cells are densely packed with little stroma; in others areas they were more widely spaced with hyalinized connective tissue and mucinous stroma. The cells have variable sized oval to elongated open-faced nuclei with one or more prominent nucleoli. Mitoses are numerous in the pictured areas. Cytoplasm is generally eosinophilic to vacuolated and streaming. Cystic degeneration was multifocal within the mass and between some lobules and nodules. There was also some chronic perivascular and nodular lymphocytic and plasma cellular inflammation within the stroma. This mass extended multifocally into the margins, appearing peeled out. Feline soft tissue sarcomas can be spontaneous, viral in origin, and they can arise in the site of a

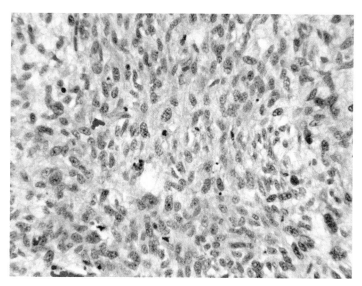

Figure 3.28 Feline fibrosarcoma biopsy. 20x.

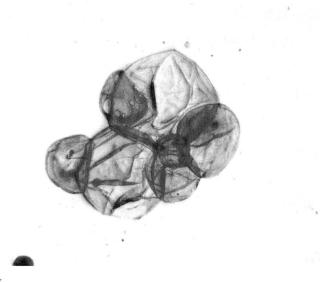

Figure 3.29 Canine lipoma FNA. 50x.

previous vaccination or injection. Viral sarcomas, which are usually seen in young cats, may be multiple, but the others are usually solitary. In any case, the cells of origin are probably primitive myofibroblasts. These tumors differentiate to various types of mesenchymal tissue, fibrosarcoma, osteosarcoma, etc. These tumors are slow to metastasize but are famous for local recurrence, even if they appear to have been completely resected. Therefore, wide resection with very careful follow-up, including specialist consultations, is usually advised.

Lipoma

Figure 3.29 shows a canine lipoma FNA. Aspirate of a soft mass on the axilla of an adult spayed female mixed breed dog revealed clumps of plump adipocytes with small nuclei. Sometimes only keratin and lipid debris will be seen if the adipocytes fail to adhere to the slide.

Figure 3.30 shows a biopsy of a canine fibrolipoma. A fluctuant subcutaneous mass was located on the plantar and lateral aspects of the right front foot of a 10-year-old spayed female Labrador Retriever. The mass consists of well-differentiated adipose tissue. The fat is dissected into smaller lobules and thick trabeculae by abundant fibrous and fibrovascular septa of varied widths. Histologic margins were indistinct, although the mass appeared circumscribed. The lesion extended into most margins, appearing peeled out. A fibrolipoma is a lipoma with a significant fibrous connective tissue component. Lipomas are considered to be benign but are sometimes multiple. Complete resection is usually curative.

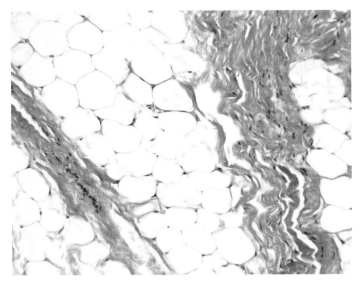

Figure 3.30 Canine fibrolipoma biopsy. 10x.

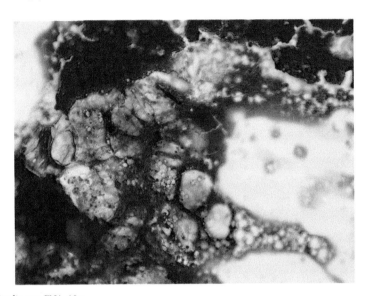

Figure 3.31 Canine infiltrative lipoma FNA. 10x.

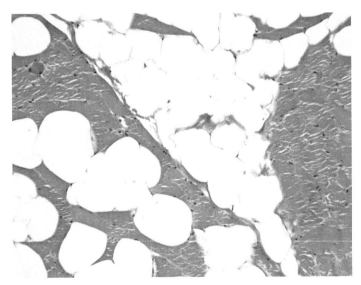

Figure 3.32 Canine infiltrative lipoma biopsy. 10x.

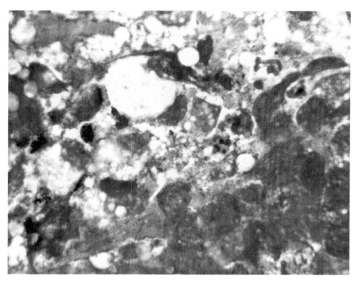

Figure 3.33 Canine liposarcoma FNA. 50x.

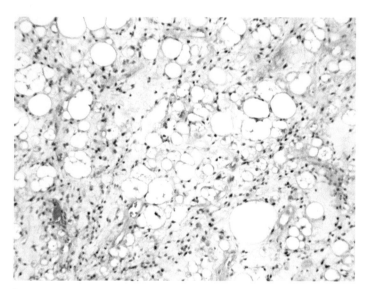

Figure 3.34 Feline liposarcoma biopsy. 10x.

Figure 3.31 shows a canine infiltrative lipoma FNA. Aspirate of a mass on the medial radius of a 13-year-old neutered male mixed breed dog yielded adipocytes and variable blood with occasional muscle or collagen fragments. When blood is present in the aspirate, biopsy is recommended to exclude a vascular tumor as the source of hemorrhage.

Figure 3.32 shows a biopsy of a canine infiltrative lipoma. A 12-year-old neutered male Bichon Frise developed what was described as a rapidly developing mass in the belly of the left biceps femoris. The adipose tissue is well differentiated. The mass infiltrates the skeletal muscle. Histologic margins were indistinct. Lipomas may be solitary or multifocal. The adipocytes are always very well differentiated, but the infiltrative variety can recur if not completely resected.

Liposarcoma

Figure 3.33 shows a canine liposarcoma FNA. Aspirate of a mass on an adult female Domestic Shorthair cat revealed many spindloid to epithelioid cells with moderate anisokaryosis and variably basophilic vacuolated cytoplasm in a background of lipid and cellular debris. The cytoplasmic vacuoles suggest the origin is from fatty tissue, but the nuclei are more typical of a sarcoma.

Figure 3.34 shows a biopsy of a feline liposarcoma. Two biopsies were submitted from a soft tissue mass on the left front leg of a 6-year-old neutered male Domestic Medium Hair cat with a previous diagnosis of panniculitis at that site. The lesion seemed to heal but then became progressive proximally. The sections consisted entirely of portions of a vaguely multilobular fatty spindle cell neoplasm with multifocal ischemia. Inflammation and infection were not

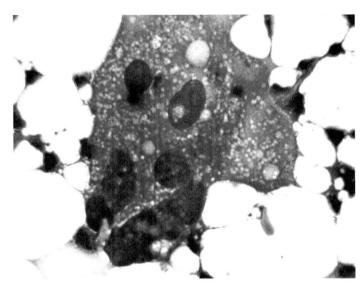

Figure 3.35 Feline synovial sarcoma FNA. 50x.

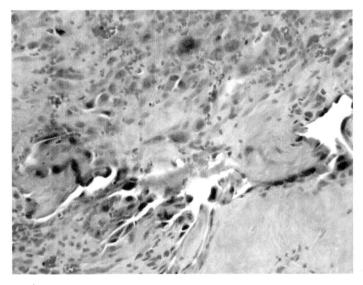

Figure 3.36 Feline synovial sarcoma biopsy. 20x.

features. The mass is comprised of small to medium polygonal and spindle cells with mild variation in nuclear size and scant cytoplasm with fat vacuoles. The intervening stroma contains abundant fat vacuoles. Most of the neoplastic cells are mononuclear. A few cells had more than one nucleus. The cells sometimes swirled around vessels. No mitoses were seen after a moderate search. The mass extended into the margins of the sections, appearing peeled out in some areas. The current mass is a soft tissue sarcoma most consistent with a liposarcoma with no evidence of panniculitis at the time of this biopsy. It is not known if the mass was near a previous injection site. Various feline soft tissue sarcomas can develop at previous injection sites with or without concurrent inflammation. Liposarcomas are likely to recur if not completely resected, and consultation with a specialist is recommended for formulation of a treatment plan that reflects the most current options. Distant metastasis is infrequent. Very careful follow-up of the surgical site was advised.

Synovial sarcoma

Figure 3.35 shows a feline synovial sarcoma FNA. Aspirate of a hock mass on an adult male Domestic Shorthair cat revealed spindloid to epithelioid cells and multinucleate cells with basophilic cytoplasm and mild to moderate nuclear pleomorphism. The primary diagnostic list includes synovial sarcoma and histiocytic sarcoma. Osteosarcoma and anaplastic fibrosarcoma can also exhibit multinucleate cells. Biopsy is necessary for definitive diagnosis.

Figure 3.36 shows a biopsy of a feline synovial sarcoma. A 12-year-old neutered male Domestic Shorthair cat developed lameness and a nonhealing oozing wound on the plantar surface of the left tarsal area that caused enough bleeding over 2 weeks to decrease the hematocrit. Subcutaneous samples were submitted. The diagnosis was pleomorphic sarcoma, most likely synovial sarcoma. The mass has a dense fibrous connective tissue stroma in some areas, and a looser edematous stroma elsewhere, with multifocal interstitial hemorrhages. The mass is comprised of pleomorphic medium to large polygonal cells that form empty branching spaces lined by one to multiple layers of crowded cells. Mitoses were seen in the neoplastic cell population at a rate of 0–1/10 HPF, at least one abnormal mitotic spindle was present, and some cells have double or multiple nuclei. There are interstitial hemorrhages, but the branching spaces were empty. Margins could not be assessed, and radiographs were not provided. The primary histologic differential was synovial sarcoma based on the biopsy material submitted, although hemangiosarcomas are relatively common on the distal limbs of cats, and they are likely to bleed. Neoplastic synovial and endothelial cells are quite similar in formalin-fixed tissues in paraffin sections. Synovial sarcomas are rarely reported in cats, and they can metastasize via both lymphatics and blood vessels. Follow-up was not available.

Additional reading

Bone lesions

Barger AM. Musculoskeletal System. In Canine and Feline Cytology; A Color Atlas and Interpretation Guide. 3rd ed. Raskin and Meyer. 2016. Elsevier. St. Louis. 353–368.

Chun R. Osteosarcoma. In Blackwell's Five-Minute Veterinary Consult: Canine and Feline. 5th ed. Tilley LP and Smith FWK, Jr. 2011. John Wiley & Sons, Inc. West Sussex, UK. 923–924.

Craig LE, Dittmer KE, Thompson KG. Bones and Joints. In Jubb, Kennedy and Palmer's Pathology of Domestic Animals. Vol 1. 6th ed. M. Grant Maxie, Editor. Elsevier. St Louis. 2016. 16–163.

Ehrhart NP, Ryan SD, Fan TM. Tumors of the Skeletal System. In Small Animal Clinical Oncology, 5th ed. Withrow and MacEwen. 2013. Elsevier. St. Louis. 463–505.

Subungual tumors

Fisher DJ. Cutaneous and Subcutaneous Lesions. In Cowell and Tyler's Diagnostic Cytology and Hematology of the Dog and Cat. 4th ed. Valenciano and Cowell. 2014. Elsevier. St. Louis. 80–109.

Gross TL, Ihrke PJ, Walder EJ, and Affolter VK. Nailbed Epithelial Tumors. In Skin Diseases of the Dog and Cat; Clinical and Histopathologic Diagnosis. 2nd ed. 2005. Blackwell Publishing. Oxford. 695–707.

Hauck ML. Tumors of the Skin and Subcutaneous Tissues. In Small Animal Clinical Oncology, 5th ed. Withrow and MacEwen. 2013. Elsevier. St. Louis. 305–320.

Mauldin EA, Peters-Kennedy JP. Integumentary System. In Jubb, Kennedy and Palmer's Pathology of Domestic Animals. Vol 1. 6th ed. M. Grant Maxie, Editor. Elsevier. St Louis. 2016. 509–736.

Raskin RE. Skin and Subcutaneous Tissue. In Canine and Feline Cytology; A Color Atlas and Interpretation Guide. 3rd ed. Raskin and Meyer. 2016. Elsevier. St. Louis. 34–90.

Melanoma

Bergman PJ, Kent MS, Farese JP. Melanoma. In Small Animal Clinical Oncology, 5th ed. Withrow and MacEwen. 2013. Elsevier. St. Louis. 321–334.

de Lorimier LP. Melanocytic Tumors, Skin and Digit. In Blackwell's Five-Minute Veterinary Consult: Canine and Feline. 5th ed. Tilley LP and Smith FWK, Jr. 2011. John Wiley & Sons, Inc. West Sussex, UK. 808–809.

Gross TL, Ihrke PJ, Walder EJ, Affolter VK. Melanocytic tumors. In Skin Diseases of the Dog and Cat; Clinical and Histopathologic Diagnosis. 2nd ed. 2005. Blackwell Publishing. Oxford. 813–836.

Squamous cell carcinoma

Gross TL, Ihrke PJ, Walder EJ, Affolter VK. Nailbed Epithelial Tumors. In Skin Diseases of the Dog and Cat; Clinical and Histopathologic Diagnosis. 2nd ed. 2005. Blackwell Publishing. Oxford. 695–707.

Wipij JM. Squamous Cell Carcinoma, Digit. Blackwell's Five-Minute Veterinary Consult: Canine and Feline. 5th ed. Tilley LP and Smith FWK, Jr. 2011. John Wiley & Sons, Inc. West Sussex, UK. 1183.

Digital skin and nail bed lesions

Fisher DJ. Cutaneous and Subcutaneous Lesions. In Cowell and Tyler's Diagnostic Cytology and Hematology of the Dog and Cat. 4th ed. Valenciano and Cowell. 2014. Elsevier. St. Louis. 80–109.

Gross TL, Ihrke PJ, Walder EJ, Affolter VK. Epidermal Tumors. In Skin Diseases of the Dog and Cat; Clinical and Histopathologic Diagnosis. 2nd ed. 2005. Blackwell Publishing. Oxford. 562–603.

Mauldin EA, Peters-Kennedy JP. Integumentary System. In Jubb, Kennedy and Palmer's Pathology of Domestic Animals. Vol 1. 6th ed. M. Grant Maxie, Editor. Elsevier. St Louis. 2016. 509–736.

Raskin RE. Skin and Subcutaneous Tissue. In Canine and Feline Cytology; A Color Atlas and Interpretation Guide. 3rd ed. Raskin and Meyer. 2016. Elsevier. St. Louis. 34–90.

Calcinosis circumscripta

Fisher DJ. Cutaneous and Subcutaneous Lesions. In Cowell and Tyler's Diagnostic Cytology and Hematology of the Dog and Cat. 4th ed. Valenciano and Cowell. 2014. Elsevier. St. Louis. 80–109.

Gross TL, Ihrke PJ, Walder EJ, Affolter VK. Degenerative, Dysplastic and Depositional Diseases of Dermal Connective Tissue. In Skin Diseases of the Dog and Cat; Clinical and Histopathologic Diagnosis. 2nd ed. 2005. Blackwell Publishing. Oxford. 373–403.

Logas DE. Dermatoses, Sterile Nodular/Granulomatous. Blackwell's Five-Minute Veterinary Consult: Canine and Feline. 5th ed. Tilley LP and Smith FWK, Jr. 2011. John Wiley & Sons, Inc. West Sussex, UK. 354–355.

Plasmacellular pododermatitis

Gross TL, Ihrke PJ, Walder EJ, Affolter VK. Nodular and Diffuse Diseases of the Dermis with Prominent Eosinophils, Neutrophils or Plasma Cells. In Skin Diseases of the Dog and Cat; Clinical and Histopathologic Diagnosis. 2nd ed. 2005. Blackwell Publishing. Oxford. 342–372.

Papilloma

Macy DW, Henry CJ. The Etiology of Cancer; Cancer Causing Viruses. In Small Animal Clinical Oncology, 5th ed. Withrow and MacEwen. 2013. Elsevier. St. Louis. 20–29.

Fibroadnexal hyperplasia

Gross TL, Ihrke PJ, Walder EJ, Affolter VK. Follicular tumors. In Skin Diseases of the Dog and Cat; Clinical and Histopathologic Diagnosis. 2nd ed. 2005. Blackwell Publishing. Oxford. 604–640.

Stromal tumors of the limb

Canine low-grade spindle cell tumor
Feline spindle cell tumor
Lipoma
Liposarcoma
Synovial sarcoma

Campbell KL. Dermatoses, Neoplastic. Blackwell's Five-Minute Veterinary Consult: Canine and Feline. 5th ed. Tilley LP and Smith FWK, Jr. 2011. John Wiley & Sons, Inc. West Sussex, UK. 350–351.

Chun R. Synovial Cell Sarcoma. In Blackwell's Five-Minute Veterinary Consult: Canine and Feline. 5th ed. Tilley LP and Smith FWK, Jr. 2011. John Wiley & Sons, Inc. West Sussex, UK. 1215.

Fisher DJ. Cutaneous and Subcutaneous Lesions. In Cowell and Tyler's Diagnostic Cytology and Hematology of the Dog and Cat. 4th ed. Valenciano and Cowell. 2014. Elsevier. St. Louis. 80–109.

Gross TL, Ihrke PJ, Walder EJ, Affolter VK. Fibrous Tumors. In Skin Diseases of the Dog and Cat; Clinical and Histopathologic Diagnosis. 2nd ed. 2005. Blackwell Publishing. Oxford. 710–734.

Gross TL, Ihrke PJ, Walder EJ, Affolter VK. Lipocytic Tumors. In Skin Diseases of the Dog and Cat; Clinical and Histopathologic Diagnosis. 2nd ed. 2005. Blackwell Publishing. Oxford. 766–777.

Gross TL, Ihrke PJ, Walder EJ, and Affolter VK. Neural and Perineural Tumors. In Skin Diseases of the Dog and Cat; Clinical and Histopathologic Diagnosis. 2nd ed. 2005. Blackwell Publishing. Oxford. 786–798.

Gross TL, Ihrke PJ, Walder EJ, Affolter VK. Mesenchymal Neoplasms and Other Tumors. In Skin Diseases of the Dog and Cat; Clinical and Histopathologic Diagnosis. 2nd ed. 2005. Blackwell Publishing. Oxford. 706–893.

Kuntz CA, Dernell WS, Powers BE, et al. JAVMA. 1997. 211:1147–1151.

Liptak JM, Forrest LJ. Soft Tissue Sarcomas. In Small Animal Clinical Oncology, 5th ed. Withrow and MacEwen. 2013. Elsevier. St. Louis. 356–380.

Mauldin EA, Peters-Kennedy JP. Integumentary System. In Jubb, Kennedy and Palmer's Pathology of Domestic Animals. Vol 1. 6th ed. M. Grant Maxie, Editor. Elsevier. St Louis. 2016. 509–736.

Mutsaers AJ. Lipoma. In Blackwell's Five-Minute Veterinary Consult: Canine and Feline. 5th ed. Tilley LP and Smith FWK, Jr. 2011. John Wiley & Sons, Inc. West Sussex, UK. 752.

Mutsaers AJ. Lipoma, Infiltrative. In Blackwell's Five-Minute Veterinary Consult: Canine and Feline. 5th ed. Tilley LP and Smith FWK, Jr. 2011. John Wiley & Sons, Inc. West Sussex, UK. 753.

Raskin RE. Skin and Subcutaneous Tissue. In Canine and Feline Cytology; A Color Atlas and Interpretation Guide. 3rd ed. Raskin and Meyer. 2016. Elsevier. St. Louis. 34–90.

4   Selected Genital and Perineal Masses

Perineal masses

Masses in the anal and perianal area originate in soft, delicate tissues, and are often recognized when they bleed or emit a malodorous discharge. Tumors of the subcutaneous glands may not be noted until after they get very large because their deep anatomic location protects them from traumatic injury while they are small.

Rectal polyp

Figure 4.1 shows a canine rectal polyp FNA. A bleeding polypoid mass was protruding from the anus of a 15-year-old male neutered mixed breed dog. Aspirate revealed clusters of plump epithelial cells with small nuclei and minimal anisokaryosis, sometimes forming columns suggestive of rectal glands. The high density of epithelial cells would not be expected in normal mucosa (e.g., rectal prolapse) and suggests that this mass has a large epithelial component. There are only low numbers of lymphocytes or eosinophils, suggesting that this mass is not an inflammatory lesion that could be treated medically. This is typical of a rectal polyp, but biopsy is recommended to exclude well-differentiated rectal carcinoma.

Figure 4.2 shows a canine rectal polyp biopsy. A bleeding mass was removed from the ventral distal colon or rectum of a 6-year-old male Dogue de Bordeaux. The mass had a micronodular to papillary surface. It is lined by crowded sometimes pseudostratified tall columnar cells. Branching glands lined by similar cells with occasional goblet cell differentiation communicate with the mucosal surface. The vascular stroma is infiltrated by lymphocytes and plasma cells, with fewer neutrophils. Mitotic figures were fairly numerous in the columnar epithelial cells. Most of these cells have basal nuclei. The stroma is somewhat congested. Margins could not be accurately assessed as the convoluted specimen was cut. These benign polypoid masses have various names: colonic or rectal papillary adenoma, adenomatous mucosal hyperplasia, mucosal polyp, etc. They may be solitary or multiple. Distal colon and rectum are the most common sites for these mucosal intestinal lesions in canines. Complete resection of individual such masses is usually curative.

Perianal gland adenoma

Figure 4.3 shows a canine perianal gland adenoma FNA. A 10-year-old intact male Anatolian Shepherd Dog presented with perianal masses. Aspirate revealed clusters of hepatoid epithelial cells with small nuclei and abundant amphophilic cytoplasm, as well as a few cells with small nuclei and scant cytoplasm presumed to be representative of the reserve cells lining the outer rim of the gland. The monomorphic nuclei and scant reserve cell population, in an intact dog that could be expected to have high hormone levels, is consistent with a diagnosis of perianal adenoma.

Figure 4.4 shows a canine perianal gland adenoma biopsy. A perianal mass was excised from a 9-year-old neutered male Boxer. The mass was fairly well circumscribed but multilobular. It is made up of large eosinophilic hepatoid cells. Tortuous trabeculae of these cells are bordered by a rim of smaller reserve cells. Perianal gland lobules on one side of the discrete mass were mildly hyperplastic. The mass appeared resected but peeled out over the deep margin. This tumor appears bland and benign histologically. Perianal gland tumors are usually benign in male dogs, and more often somewhat aggressive in females. They are hormone responsive and frequently multiple (thus the usual recommendation for castration of males).

Atlas for the Diagnosis of Tumors in the Dog and Cat, First Edition. Anita R. Kiehl and Maron Brown Calderwood Mays.
© 2016 John Wiley & Sons, Inc. Published 2016 by John Wiley & Sons, Inc.

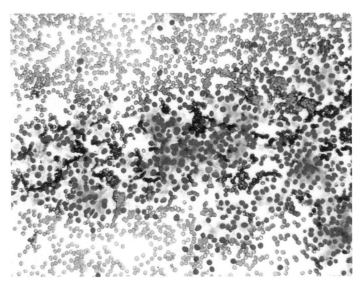

Figure 4.1 Canine rectal polyp FNA. 10x.

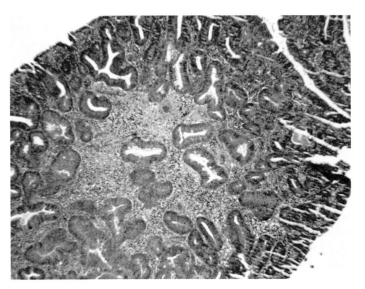

Figure 4.2 Canine rectal polyp biopsy. 4x.

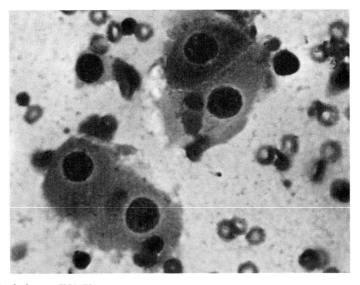

Figure 4.3 Canine perianal gland adenoma FNA. 50x.

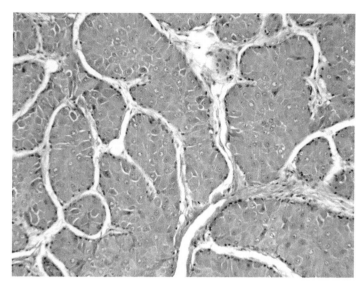

Figure 4.4 Canine perianal gland adenoma biopsy. 10x.

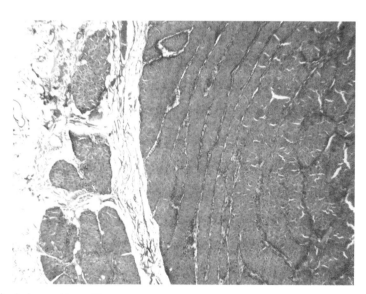

Figure 4.5 Canine perianal gland adenoma biopsy. 10x.

Figure 4.5 shows a biopsy of a canine perianal gland adenoma. A 10-year-old spayed female German Shepherd Dog exhibited a perianal mass, which on excision was revealed to be a circumscribed proliferation of densely packed perianal gland epithelium (large mass on the right side of the photomicrograph) with a typical reserve cell lining. Examination at 10x reveals hyperplastic perianal glands (the multiple smaller masses on the left side of the photomicrograph) in the tissue surrounding the mass. In a spayed female, there may be ongoing adrenal androgenic hormone stimulation of these adjacent glands, which may result in growth of additional masses. This tumor appears well differentiated, and complete excision of the larger mass may be curative, but since additional growths may arise from the adjacent plump glands, periodic rechecks are advised.

Perianal gland carcinoma

Figure 4.6 shows a perianal gland tumor FNA. A 6-year-old neutered male mixed breed dog presented with a perineal mass. There are clusters of hepatoid epithelial cells with moderately pleomorphic nuclei and abundant amphophilic cytoplasm. In addition, and of diagnostic significance, there are increased numbers of smaller reserve cells (arrow) with small nuclei and scant to moderate cytoplasm. This increased reserve cell component can be seen with perianal gland carcinoma, a more aggressive tumor type, and since the dog is neutered with presumably a low testosterone level, biopsy is indicated for prognosis.

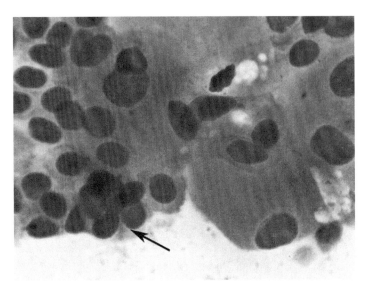

Figure 4.6 Perianal gland tumor FNA. 50x.

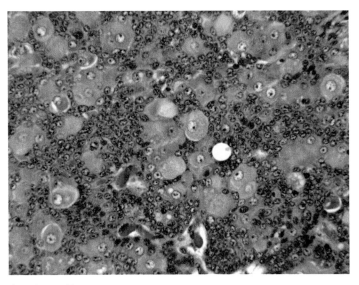

Figure 4.7 Canine perianal gland carcinoma. 20x.

Figure 4.7 shows a canine perianal gland carcinoma. A biopsy of a perianal mass from an 11-year-old spayed female Border Collie cross was submitted. The surface was ulcerated and the mass had a multifocally inflamed somewhat fibrous stroma. Lobules are composed of moderately pleomorphic enlarged hepatoid cells in some areas, but in most areas the mass is composed of lobules of smaller epithelial cells with less cytoplasm, moderate variation in cell and nuclear size, and a mitotic rate in the immature cell population of 0–3/HPF. The mass extended into the deep and one lateral margin of the specimen. Most canine perianal gland tumors are benign in behavior, although they are frequently multiple, but the cells comprising this one have malignant histologic features and an increased mitotic rate. Malignant varieties can recur if not completely resected, and they can also metastasize via lymphatics, so consultation with a specialist and careful follow-up was advised.

Anal sac apocrine gland carcinoma

Figure 4.8 shows a canine anal sac apocrine gland carcinoma FNA. An adult female dog presented with a circumscribed mass lateral to the anus. The mass was aspirated and yielded sheets and ribbons of small apocrine type epithelial cells with mild to rare moderate anisokaryosis and scant to moderate lightly basophilic cytoplasm. The cells sometimes formed ribbons and acinar-like structures. This feature is typical of anal sac apocrine gland carcinoma. This tumor may

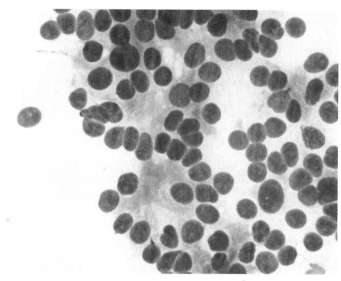

Figure 4.8 Canine anal sac apocrine gland carcinoma FNA. 40x.

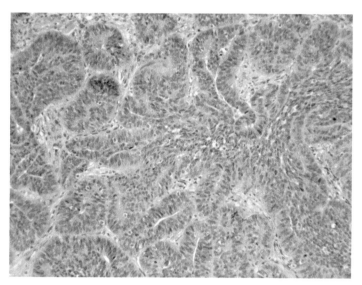

Figure 4.9 Canine anal sac apocrine gland adenocarcinoma biopsy. 10x.

cause hypercalcemia, a paraneoplastic syndrome, which if present, alerts the practitioner that the benign cytologic appearance of this FNA may mask an underlying aggressive tumor type, and there is a need for early complete excision of the mass with biopsy documentation of wide clean margins.

Figure 4.9. There was a mass in the anal sac wall of a 10-year-old neutered male King Charles Cavalier Spaniel. The anal sac was lined by well-differentiated stratified squamous epithelium. In the wall is a multilobular/multinodular epithelial neoplasm comprised of somewhat pleomorphic medium-sized polygonal, cuboidal, and sometimes more squamoid epithelial cells that line acini and branching tubules. There is some variation in cell and nuclear size, and mitotic figures can be found in this cell population. Chronic inflammation was noted around the affected anal sac and multifocally surrounded the adjacent mass. The mass appeared completely resected. This is an adenocarcinoma of the apocrine glands that surround the anal sac. These tumors can recur even after complete resection, and they can also metastasize to the sacral, sublumbar, and inguinal lymph nodes, and then to more distant sites. This is the canine neoplasm most often associated with paraneoplastic hypercalcemia. Complete resection of the neoplasm corrects the hypercalcemia, but the serum calcium levels should be monitored. Recurrence of the hypercalcemia could indicate tumor recurrence or a metastasis. This tumor is more common in females than in males, and affected patients are usually elderly.

Masses of the external genitalia

Proliferative lesions of the haired skin and mucocutaneous junction of the vulva, penile sheath, and scrotum include epithelial tumors such as papilloma and squamous cell carcinoma, vascular tumors such as hemangioma and hemangiosarcoma, and round cell tumors such as mast cell tumor (MCT) and transmissible venereal tumor (TVT).

Transmissible venereal tumor

Figure 4.10 shows a canine TVT FNA. A 3-year-old neutered male Bulldog presented with a mass on the penis. This shows numerous round cells with prominent nucleoli and occasional small cytoplasmic vacuoles typical of TVT.

Figure 4.11 shows a biopsy of a canine vaginal TVT. A 10-year-old intact female Boxer was presented with a bleeding vaginal tumor. It was a 4.7 × 2.4 × 2.0 cm tan/brown irregular soft tissue mass without distinct gross margins. It was ulcerated, inflamed, and multilobular, multinodular, and multicentric in the mucosa and submucosa of the vagina at the time of presentation. This is a round cell neoplasm most consistent with canine transmissible venereal tumor. The mass is comprised of sheets of pleomorphic yet somewhat homogeneous medium-sized round and polygonal cells with a central or eccentric nucleolus and scant to moderate faintly granular eosinophilic cytoplasm,

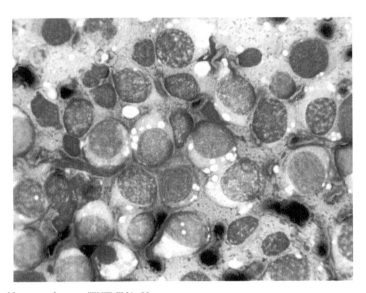

Figure 4.10 Canine transmissible venereal tumor (TVT) FNA. 50x.

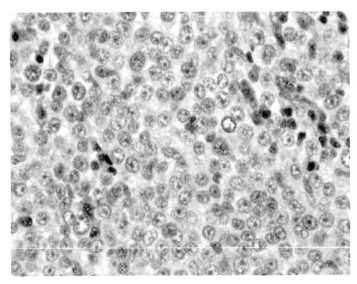

Figure 4.11 Canine vaginal TVT biopsy. 40x.

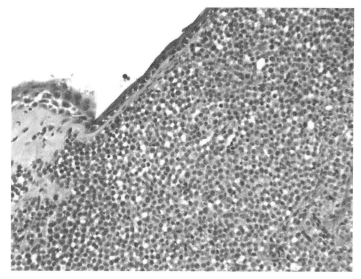

Figure 4.12 Canine vaginal TVT biopsy. 10x.

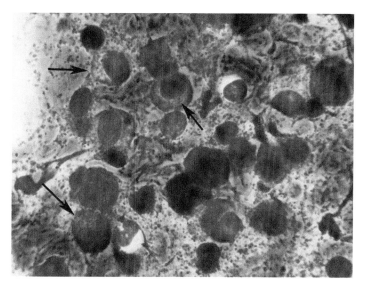

Figure 4.13 Canine scrotal mast cell tumor from impression. 50x.

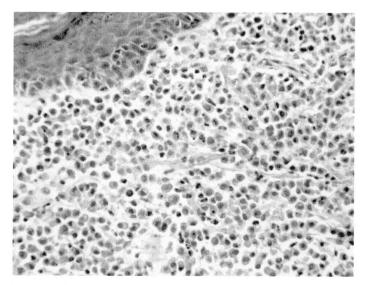

Figure 4.14 Canine scrotal grade 2/low-grade mast cell tumor biopsy. 20x.

often with distinct cell borders. Moderate numbers of mitoses were seen in this cell population. The mass had a rather narrow base, and margins available for examination on the sections were clean. These tumors may be solitary or multicentric within the vagina. Most of them eventually spontaneously regress. Disseminating metastasis is rare. This is a sexually transmitted neoplasm.

Figure 4.12 shows a biopsy of a canine vaginal TVT. A 3-year-old spayed female mixed breed dog presented with a mass at the mucocutaneous junction of the vulva. This low power view of a canine TVT reveals sheets of round cells that could be mistaken for a mast cell tumor with routine stains. Giemsa stain or Toluidine Blue special stain (see Chapter 8) might be helpful to look for mast cell granules if there is question as to the tumor type. The clinical history of an expanding mass on a genital mucocutaneous surface is a significant diagnostic feature of this lesion. Metastatic disease in rare individuals can result in diagnosis of this tumor at other sites.

Mast cell tumor

Figure 4.13 shows a canine scrotal mast cell tumor. Impression of a mass on the scrotum of an adult intact male Bulldog revealed sheets and clusters of variably granulated mast cells in a background of blood. Finding dense clusters of well-granulated mast cells is diagnostic for mast cell tumor. Care must be taken to identify at least some cells with granules contained within an intact cytoplasmic membrane (arrows), because free cellular debris can sometimes mimic mast cell granules, and irritation at this site often causes ulceration and exudation.

Figure 4.14 shows a biopsy of a canine scrotal grade 2/low-grade mast cell tumor. A rescued 2-year-old male Boxer was found to have a raised 0.5 cm skin mass on the left scrotum. Fine needle aspirate yielded mast cells, so castration and scrotal ablation were performed. The mass is comprised of variably granulated mast cells in sheets and narrow cords. There is mild variation in nuclear size. MI = 0/10 HPF, but scattered cells had double nuclei. Individual eosinophils accompany the mast cells. There was a much smaller separate shallower but similar nodule immediately adjacent to the primary raised mass. Both appeared completely resected. There is an increased incidence of mast cell tumors in Boxers. Canine mast cell tumors on the scrotum are sometimes poorly differentiated, but this one is still well differentiated. These tumors are capable of local recurrence, multicentric appearance, and metastasis via lymphatics.

Additional reading

Uzal FA, Plattner BL, Hostetter JM. Integumentary System. In Jubb, Kennedy and Palmer's Pathology of Domestic Animals. Vol 1. 6th ed. M. Grant Maxie, Editor. Elsevier. St Louis. 2016. 509–736.

Perineal masses

Rectal polyp
Pope ER. Rectoanal Polyps. In Blackwell's Five-Minute Veterinary Consult: Canine and Feline. 5th ed. Tilley LP and Smith FWK, Jr. 2011. John Wiley & Sons, Inc. West Sussex, UK. 1087.

Perianal gland adenoma
Perianal gland carcinoma
Gross TL, Ihrke PJ, Walder EJ, Affolter VK. Sebaceous Tumors. In Skin Diseases of the Dog and Cat; Clinical and Histopathologic Diagnosis. 2nd ed. 2005. Blackwell Publishing. Oxford. 641–654.
Turek MM, Withrow SJ. Perianal Tumors. In Small Animal Clinical Oncology, 5th ed. Withrow and MacEwen. 2013. Elsevier. St. Louis. 423–431.

Anal sac apocrine gland carcinoma
Garrett LD. Adenocarcinoma, Anal Sac. In Blackwell's Five-Minute Veterinary Consult: Canine and Feline. 5th ed. Tilley LP and Smith FWK, Jr. 2011. John Wiley & Sons, Inc. West Sussex, UK. 24.

Masses of the external genitalia

Lawrence JA, Saba CF. Tumors of the Male Reproductive System. In In Small Animal Clinical Oncology, 5th ed. Withrow and MacEwen. 2013. Elsevier. St. Louis. 557–571.

Transmissible venereal tumor

Chun R. Transmissible Venereal Tumor. In Blackwell's Five-Minute Veterinary Consult: Canine and Feline. 5th ed. Tilley LP and Smith FWK, Jr. 2011. John Wiley & Sons, Inc. West Sussex, UK. 1249.

Gross TL, Ihrke PJ, Walder EJ, Affolter VK. Other Mesenchymal Tumors. In Skin Diseases of the Dog and Cat; Clinical and Histopathologic Diagnosis. 2nd ed. 2005. Blackwell Publishing. Oxford. 797–812.

Woods JP. Canine Transmissible Venereal Tumor. In Small Animal Clinical Oncology, 5th ed. Withrow and MacEwen. 2013. Elsevier. St. Louis. 692–696.

Mast cell tumor

Gross TL, Ihrke PJ, Walder EJ, and Affolter VK. Mast Cell Tumors. In Skin Diseases of the Dog and Cat; Clinical and Histopathologic Diagnosis. 2nd ed. 2005. Blackwell Publishing. Oxford. 853–865.

5 Selected Lesions of the Skin and Subcutis of the Trunk

Mass lesions of the dorsal trunk

Circumscribed, superficial, occasionally cystic masses are common in the dog and cat. FNA can reveal cells that are clearly neoplastic and aggressive, such as mast cells or carcinoma cells, but often the sample consists of mostly keratin debris and a few scattered diagnostic cells. Biopsy is necessary for definitive diagnosis and evaluation of margins. Only biopsy can identify the type of cyst because the cyst type depends on the morphology of the cyst wall, and cell wall morphology is not retained with FNA. Biopsy is helpful for prognosis because cystic adnexal tumors, even if benign, can rupture and release keratin into the adjacent tissue, causing an intense inflammatory response and chronic draining tract. It can be useful for prognosis to know if there was complete excision of the debris because incomplete excision can result in chronic draining tracts. Biopsy can sometimes lead to a preliminary diagnosis of metabolic disease such as Cushing's disease, based on morphologic changes specific to the disease process, and appropriate diagnostic procedures can be initiated. Excision of cystic adnexal tumors is usually curative, but malignant tumors can arise de novo or from chronic benign lesions, and margin evaluation is important.

Calcinosis cutis

Figure 5.1 shows a clinical presentation of a dermal flank lesion. This dog has the alopecia and pot-bellied appearance of hyperadrenocorticism (Cushing's disease). There are occasional crusted plaques in the skin.

Figure 5.2 shows a canine calcinosis cutis FNA. Aspiration of a thickened skin lesion on the flank of a 14-year-old female Bulldog with Cushing's disease reveals scattered neutrophils and macrophages with occasional multinucleate giant cells containing amorphous basophilic material suggestive of mineralized debris.

Figure 5.3 shows a biopsy of a canine calcinosis cutis. An adult female spayed mixed breed dog presented with multiple skin plaques, some ulcerated and bleeding. Biopsy revealed multiple sites of mineralized collagen surrounded by walls of fibrosis-containing macrophages and neutrophils, changes suggestive of hypercortisolism. Evaluation of cortisol levels before and after administration of dexamethasone and adrenocorticotrophic hormone confirmed the suspected hypercortisolism.

Follicular cyst

Figure 5.4 shows a gross tissue cross section of a hip skin mass revealing a cystic dermal lesion.

Figure 5.5 shows a canine dermal cyst FNA. Aspiration of a freely movable dermal hip mass on a 14-year-old male Shih Tzu dog reveals abundant keratin flakes in variable blood. This suggests an adnexal cyst or cystic tumor.

Figure 5.6 shows a biopsy of a canine follicular cyst. Excisional biopsy of a dermal cystic mass on the hip of a 2-year-old Poodle mixed breed dog reveals a dilated hair follicle lined by attenuated squamous epithelium and filled with keratin. This is a benign lesion, and complete excision should be curative. If the cyst ruptures prior to excision, release of keratin into the adjacent stroma can cause an intense inflammatory response due to the foreign body effect of the free keratin. This can lead to a draining tract that requires wider tissue margins, so removal of these lesions while small and intact is recommended.

Atlas for the Diagnosis of Tumors in the Dog and Cat, First Edition. Anita R. Kiehl and Maron Brown Calderwood Mays.
© 2016 John Wiley & Sons, Inc. Published 2016 by John Wiley & Sons, Inc.

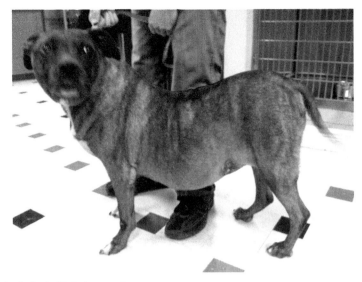

Figure 5.1 Clinical photograph of a flank skin lesion on a dog.

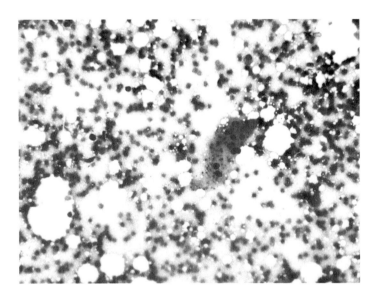

Figure 5.2 Canine calcinosis cutis FNA. 10x.

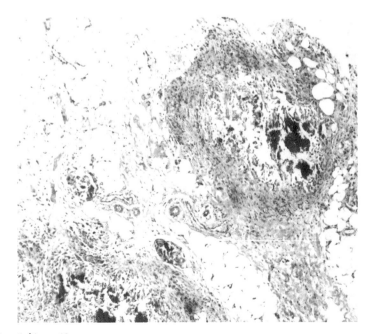

Figure 5.3 Canine calcinosis cutis biopsy. 10x.

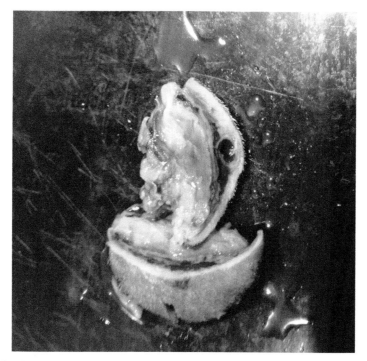

Figure 5.4 Gross section of a hip skin mass with a cystic dermal lesion.

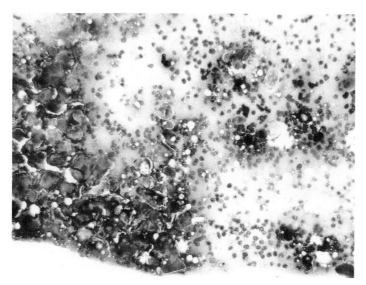

Figure 5.5 Canine dermal cyst FNA. 10x.

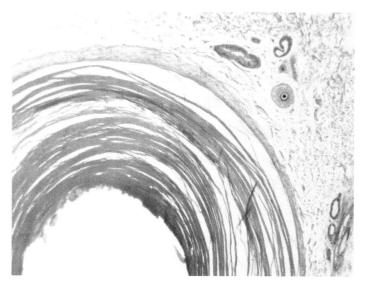

Figure 5.6 Canine follicular cyst biopsy. 2.5x.

Cystic adnexal tumors—trichoepithelioma, keratoacanthoma

Figure 5.7 shows a canine cystic adnexal tumor FNA. Aspirate of cystic adnexal tumors such as trichoepithelioma, pilomatricoma, and keratoacanthoma (intradermal cornifying epithelioma) can yield a mixed picture of keratin debris (arrow), sheets of small epithelial cells with monomorphic small round nuclei and scant pale cytoplasm (arrowhead), and clumps of variably pigmented to golden refractile material suggestive of follicle root sheath material.

Figure 5.8 shows a canine trichoepithelioma biopsy. A 4-year-old spayed female Golden Retriever was presented with a 2-month history of a rapidly growing nodule on her side. A 1.9 x 1.5 x 1.3 cm portion of skin with a raised nodular mass was submitted, and a representative central section was processed. The mass was comprised of multiple islands of neoplastic basaloid cells resembling those of the hair follicles, abortive branching follicular structures, and larger cysts lined by similar cells with multifocal squamous differentiation or abrupt keratinization. The cysts and follicular structures are filled with a combination of lamellar and amorphous keratin and clumps of ghost epithelial cells. The mass rose above the skin surface but also involved the superficial subcutis. The mass extended focally just into the deep margin on one side within the subcutis. Other margins were clean. This is a trichoepithelioma, a tumor of hair follicle origin. This tumor type is usually benign and solitary but may be multiple in certain breeds of dogs. These tumors can recur if not completely resected.

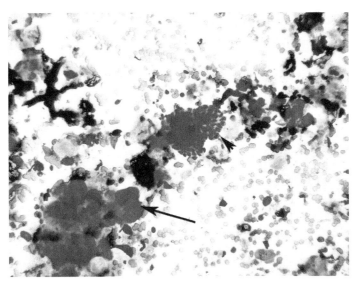

Figure 5.7 Canine cystic adnexal tumor FNA. 10x.

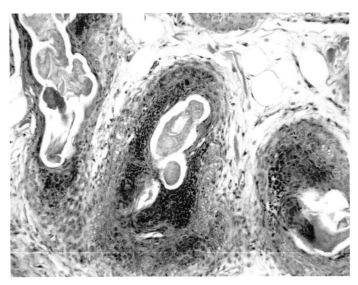

Figure 5.8 Canine trichoepithelioma biopsy. 10x.

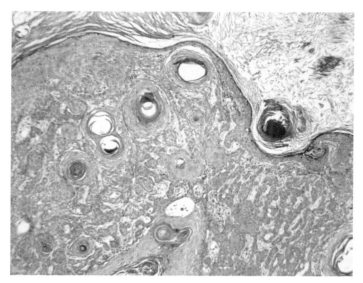

Figure 5.9 Canine infundibular keratinizing acanthoma biopsy. 4x.

Figure 5.9 shows a canine infundibular keratinizing acanthoma, right lumbar region biopsy. This tumor is also called intracutaneous cornifying epithelioma and keratoacanthoma. It is from a 10-year-old spayed female Akita mix. It is a fairly well-circumscribed nodular dermal mass with a central cystic space filled with keratin. The central cyst is surrounded by a thick irregular wall of fairly well-differentiated stratified squamous epithelium. Additional smaller horn cysts are found throughout the wall. There was granulomatous inflammation within the central keratin-filled cyst, and leakage of keratin had incited inflammation and fibrosis peripheral to the mass. Margins were clean. This type of tumor is usually benign and solitary. A central cystic cavity often communicates by a pore with the skin surface. These lesions may be multiple in Norwegian Elkhounds, and occasionally in other breeds.

Apocrine adenoma

Figure 5.10 shows a feline apocrine gland proliferation FNA. Aspiration of a dermal mass on an adult male Persian cat yielded clusters and chains of moderate to large epithelial cells with mild anisokaryosis, abundant lightly basophilic cytoplasm, and occasional intracellular blue/gray material presumed to be apocrine gland secretory product. There may be variable blood and mixed inflammatory infiltrates.

Figure 5.11 shows a feline apocrine ductal adenoma biopsy. This mass is from between the shoulders of a 14-year-old Domestic Longhair cat. The mass was cellular but had a dense moderately cellular fibrovascular stroma in some areas, and chronic lymphocytic and plasma cellular inflammation around the periphery and between some lobules and nodules. There were some cysts (not shown), and the cysts were often empty, but sometimes contained pale eosinophilic secretion. The branching tubules and ductules are mostly lined by a double row of cells similar to the linings of apocrine ducts. Stromal invasion and intralymphatic spread were not seen around the periphery of the mass. Scattered pigment-laden macrophages in the stroma were thought to indicate previous leakage of secretion. Margins were clean. This is a neoplasm of apocrine gland origin. Apocrine tumors are usually solitary, occasionally multiple. The cells comprising this one appear fairly bland and benign, and resection was expected to be curative.

Apocrine and sebaceous carcinoma

Figure 5.12 shows a feline adnexal carcinoma FNA. Aspiration of a dermal mass on the rump of an adult neutered male Domestic Shorthair cat yielded large epithelioid cells with marked anisokaryosis, multiple giant nuclei, and basophilic variably vacuolated cytoplasm. An atypical mitotic figure was seen (arrow). It is not possible to determine the cell of origin from cytologic exam as the cells are anaplastic and undifferentiated, but a preliminary diagnosis of carcinoma can be made. Biopsy is necessary to determine the tumor type.

Figure 5.13 shows a biopsy of a canine apocrine ductal carcinoma. A 6-1/2-year-old neutered male Labrador Retriever developed an ulcerated mass involving the dermis and subcutis of the left dorsal thorax with encroachment on underlying skeletal muscle. The mass had a moderate fibrovascular stroma. It is comprised of pleomorphic small, medium, and sometimes fairly large polygonal, cuboidal, and occasionally low columnar epithelial cells that form

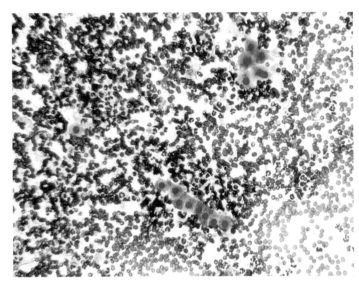

Figure 5.10 Feline apocrine gland proliferation FNA.

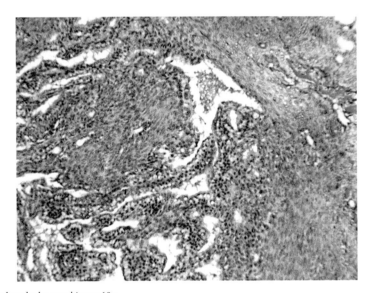

Figure 5.11 Feline apocrine ductal adenoma biopsy. 10x.

branching tubules and ductules often lined by a double row of crowded cells similar to the ducts of normal apocrine glands. There was multifocal squamous differentiation, as occurs at the junctions of the apocrine ducts with the hair follicles. The squamous cells were also pleomorphic, with multifocal apoptosis and necrosis. Mitoses were seen in the apocrine cell population at a rate of up to 3/HPF. Mitotic figures were also found in the squamous cell population. The mass was not well circumscribed, and there were small nodules peripheral to the main mass. However, definitive intralymphatic embolization was not seen. Margins were clean, but the deep margin was narrow. This is a malignant neoplasm of apocrine duct origin. These tumors can recur even if completely resected, and they can also metastasize to draining lymph nodes and the lungs. Canine apocrine tumors are sometimes multicentric, as well.

Sebaceous carcinoma
Figure 5.14 shows a canine sebocytic sebaceous carcinoma, right flank biopsy. A 12-year-old neutered male Shepherd cross developed a pigmented raised skin mass on the right flank. The surface was ulcerated with suppurative granulation tissue proliferating in the ulcer bed, maturing to a fairly dense fibrous connective tissue stroma. The mass was rather poorly circumscribed and was multilobular/multinodular. The lobules are comprised of moderately pleomorphic medium to large polygonal cells with moderate variation in nuclear size, at least one prominent nucleolus, and a moderate amount of vacuolated cytoplasm. The cells have distinct cell borders. Cells with more

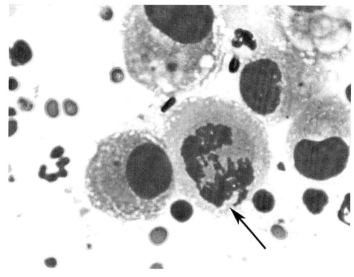

Figure 5.12 Feline adnexal carcinoma FNA. 50x.

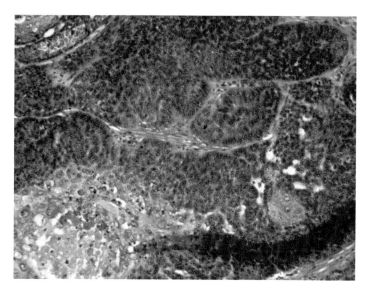

Figure 5.13 Canine apocrine ductal carcinoma biopsy. 10x.

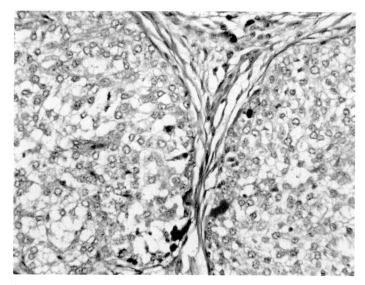

Figure 5.14 Canine sebocytic sebaceous carcinoma biopsy. 20x.

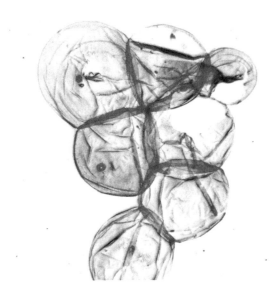

Figure 5.15 Canine lipoma FNA. 50x.

Figure 5.16 Canine subcutaneous lipoma biopsy. 10x.

than one nucleus are present. Mitoses were seen at a rate of 0–2/HPF. Intralymphatic embolization was not seen at the level examined. However, there were stromal invasions along the periphery of the mass. Margins were clean. These tumors sometimes recur even if completely resected. They are usually slow to metastasize, but can spread to regional lymph nodes.

Lipoma

The most common tumor seen in the subcutis is the lipoma. This tumor type is generally benign but can get very large and interfere with normal limb function. FNA will usually result in a preliminary diagnosis that will allow the surgeon to take reasonable margins based on the tumor type. Injection reactions are a common cause of a transient subcutaneous mass that can feel like a lipoma and usually do not require excision in dogs. Occasionally FNA reveals a more aggressive tumor such as a sarcoma or a mast cell tumor. Obtaining a preliminary diagnosis by FNA allows for presurgical planning for adequate margins and is an important part of clinical management.

Figure 5.15 shows a canine lipoma FNA. Aspiration of soft, deep dermal and subcutaneous masses can yield clusters of plump adipocytes with scant slender nuclei. This is typical of fat or lipoma.

Figure 5.16 shows a canine subcutaneous lipoma, trunk biopsy. A 7-1/2-year-old neutered male Labrador Retriever had multiple subcutaneous fatty tumors. The mass submitted consists of well-differentiated adipose tissue. The mass

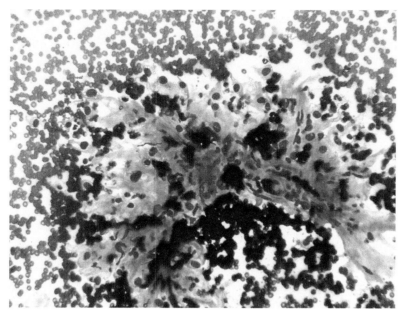

Figure 5.17 Canine spindle cell proliferation FNA. 10x.

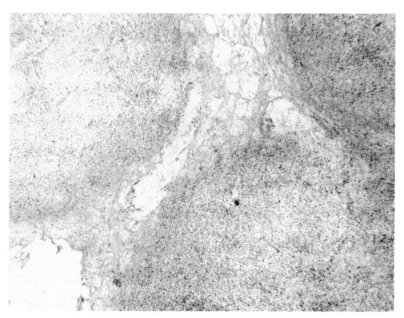

Figure 5.18 Canine reactive fibroplasias FNA. 2.5x.

was somewhat circumscribed but not encapsulated. Histologic margins were indistinct. Lipomas are considered benign but they are sometimes multiple, and they occasionally behave in an infiltrative manner.

Canine well-differentiated spindle cell proliferation

Figure 5.17 shows a canine spindle cell proliferation FNA. This aspirate from a dorsal lumbar subcutaneous firm mass on a 12-year-old female mixed breed dog revealed blood and clusters of slender spindle cells with small ovoid to round nuclei sometimes associated with an eosinophilic matrix. There were slightly increased neutrophils and a few macrophages in some areas. This indicates a spindle cell proliferation but does not distinguish reactive hyperplasia from low-grade neoplasia. Biopsy is necessary for definitive diagnosis and prognosis.

Figure 5.18 shows a biopsy of a canine spindle cell proliferation in reaction to an injection. This 1-year-old male neutered mixed breed dog presented with an enlarging mass on the dorsal lumbar region. Excision and biopsy revealed

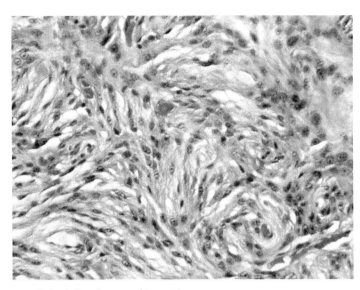

Figure 5.19 Canine subcutaneous grade 1 spindle cell sarcoma biopsy. 20x.

a cavitated region in the deep dermis surrounded by somewhat nodular proliferations of well-differentiated spindle cells with occasional infiltrates of neutrophils and macrophages, a finding compatible with a reactive response to an injury. The lesion was circumscribed, but inflammation extended to some margins. A history of recent vaccination at this site was noted.

Figure 5.19 shows a canine subcutaneous grade 1 spindle cell sarcoma, suspected neurofibrosarcoma, left thorax biopsy. A subcutaneous mass was removed from the left thorax of a spayed female Labrador Retriever of unknown age. Within the tissue was a multilobular mass of neoplastic polygonal and plump spindle cells. These cells are organized in interlacing bundles, swirls, and herringbone patterns. Some areas are very cellular with little stroma; in other areas the cells are more loosely arranged with moderate amounts of collagen. The cells have oval to elongated nuclei with one or two nucleoli. Mitoses occurred in low to moderate numbers, but occasional multinucleated cells were noted. Cytoplasm is generally eosinophilic and streaming with indistinct cell borders. Margins were clean but as narrow as 0.2 mm fat. Scores: Differentiation, suspected nerve sheath origin = 2; mitoses, MI = 3/10 HPF = 1; necrosis, none = 1. Total = 4. Grade 1. The spindle cell tumors are difficult to differentiate by light microscopy. The most common differentials include fibrosarcoma, canine hemangiopericytoma, and tumors of nerve or nerve sheath origin (neurofibroma, neurofibrosarcoma, schwannoma). Nerve sheath origin was suspected in this case because of proliferative pattern and cytologic features. However, all of these tumors are slow to metastasize but are famous for local recurrence. Therefore, radical resection and careful follow-up are usually recommended and pre-surgical consultation with oncology and surgical specialists is suggested.

Canine spindle cell tumor, mid grade

Figure 5.20 shows a canine mid-grade spindle cell tumor FNA. This proliferation of plump spindle cells was aspirated from a rapidly growing subcutaneous mass on the back of a 12-year-old male Labrador Retriever. The spindle cells are moderately pleomorphic with moderate anisokaryosis, occasional prominent nucleoli, and basophilic wispy cytoplasm. They are clearly spindle shaped, and a preliminary diagnosis of spindle cell tumor was made with recommendation for biopsy with wide margins.

Figure 5.21 shows a canine subcutaneous grade 2 spindle cell sarcoma, suspected neurofibrosarcoma, left shoulder biopsy. An 11-year-old female Boxer had multiple medical problems, one of which was a dermal/subcutaneous mass on the left shoulder. This mass is very similar to the grade 1 spindle cell sarcoma described immediately above. Mitoses were seen in low numbers, but some cells had multiple nuclei. Focal ischemic necrosis was noted within the mass, with an interstitial hemorrhage in the necrotic area. The mass involved the deep dermis and subcutis. It appeared partially peeled out along the deep border and extended focally into the cauterized margin of the superficial subcutis on one side. Scores: Differentiation, suspected nerve sheath origin = 2; mitoses, 1/10 HPF = 1; necrosis, < 50% = 2. Total = 5. Grade 2. Nerve sheath origin was suspected in this case because of cytologic features and proliferative pattern. Necrosis in this tumor raises the score to grade 2.

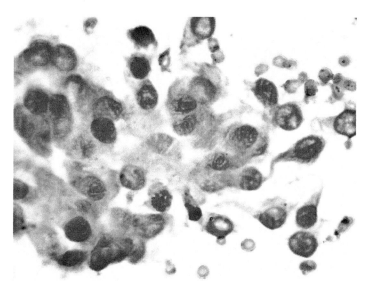

Figure 5.20 Canine mid-grade spindle cell tumor FNA. 50x.

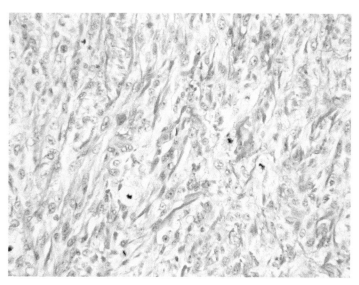

Figure 5.21 Canine subcutaneous grade 2 spindle cell sarcoma biopsy. 20x.

Canine spindle cell tumor, high grade

Figure 5.22 shows a canine high-grade spindle cell tumor FNA. Aspiration of a subcutaneous mass on the shoulder of an adult spayed female mixed breed dog revealed a pleomorphic population of spindloid to epithelioid cells with marked anisokaryosis, prominent nucleoli, and basophilic, occasionally finely vacuolated cytoplasm sometimes associated with eosinophilic matrix. There are spindle cells present, but many of the cells exhibit rounded cytoplasmic borders suggesting loss of normal cellular architecture and possibly predictive of impaired cellular adhesion.

Figure 5.23 shows a canine high-grade spindle cell tumor biopsy. This 5-year-old Puggle presented for a rapidly growing subcutaneous mass. There are proliferating epithelioid to spindloid cells infiltrating around and expanding the stroma between muscle bundles. There is moderate nuclear pleomorphism at this site. The cells are not clearly spindloid, and it is difficult to identify the cell type in this area. Scattered mitotic figures are seen and there are occasional foci of necrosis throughout the lesion. The infiltrative, poorly differentiated nature of the cells along with a mitotic index greater than 10/10 HPF and scattered necrosis indicates a high-grade soft tissue sarcoma. Immunohistochemistry could be used to identify the cell type for a more definitive diagnosis. The lesion extended to all margins and without additional wider excision for clean margins, would be expected to regrow in a progressively more aggressive manner.

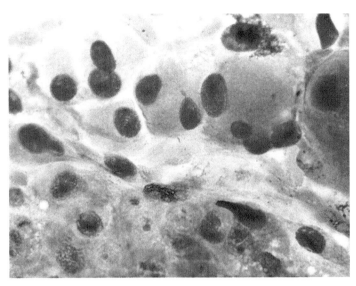

Figure 5.22 Canine high-grade spindle cell tumor FNA. 50x.

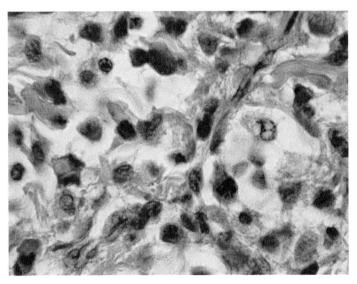

Figure 5.23 Canine high-grade spindle cell tumor biopsy. 40x.

Figure 5.24 shows a biopsy of a canine spindle cell tumor. Excisional biopsies of soft tissue sarcomas are sometimes presented with a history of "the mass shelled out cleanly." This tumor type will follow fascial planes and send out small projections into adjacent tissues. The "shelling out" is merely the separation of those fascial planes and does not necessarily indicate a boundary between affected and normal tissue. Since normal tissue can be somewhat resistant to separation along fascial planes, that ease of separation may indicate compromised tissue and is an indication for wider excision into adjacent normal tissue. Advanced imaging techniques such as computed tomography (CT) or magnetic resonance imaging (MRI) may be most helpful to determine the extent of the tumor and the location of normal tissue. Consultation with specialists in oncology and surgery is recommended for these types of tumors because complete excision is of great prognostic importance.

Feline spindle cell tumor
Feline spindle cell tumors of all types are locally invasive and often extend far beyond the borders of a grossly visible mass. Regrowth is common, often in a progressively more aggressive fashion. Consultation with a specialist is recommended prior to initiating treatment of this tumor type.

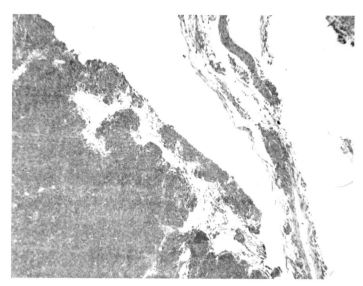

Figure 5.24 Canine spindle cell tumor biopsy. 2.5x.

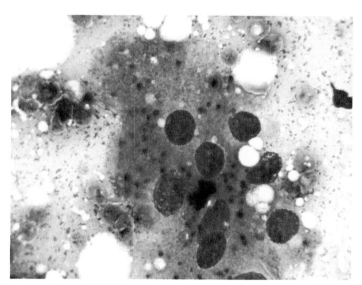

Figure 5.25 Feline spindle cell tumor FNA. 50x.

Figure 5.25 shows a feline spindle cell tumor FNA. Aspiration of a subcutaneous mass on the trunk or a hind limb will sometimes yield multinucleate giant cells, of macrophage lineage, containing basophilic amorphous material that is postulated by some to be vaccine adjuvant. Vaccination in cats, especially rabies vaccination, has historically been associated with formation of aggressive soft tissue sarcoma at the vaccination site in up to 0.1% of vaccinated cats. The presence of a cell such as this, at a vaccination site with a progressively enlarging mass at least 4 weeks post-vaccination, is an indication for immediate further therapy. Identification of this cell is not diagnostic for neoplasia, but this type of cell is often present in areas of vaccination-associated sarcoma. Consultation with a specialist is recommended in order to utilize the most current diagnostic and treatment options available.

Figure 5.26 shows a feline spindle cell tumor FNA. Aspirate of a subcutaneous mass on the trunk of a 12-year-old cat yielded clusters of plump spindle cells with moderate anisokaryosis, small nucleoli, and spindled lightly basophilic cytoplasm in variable eosinophilic matrix. These cells are suggestive of, but not diagnostic for, spindle cell neoplasia, if there is no evidence of traumatic injury or recent vaccination. Reactive fibroplasia can sometimes have this appearance, so it is important to exclude traumatic injury when considering the etiology of this type of mass. Biopsy is suggested for definitive diagnosis if the lesion persists.

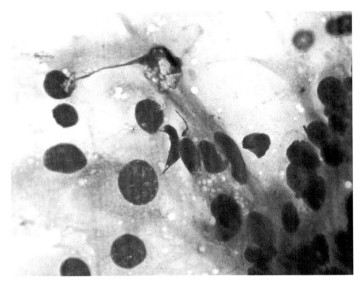

Figure 5.26 Feline spindle cell tumor FNA. 50x.

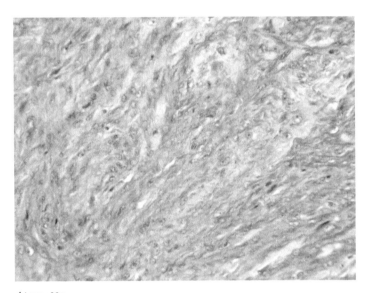

Figure 5.27 Feline fibrosarcoma biopsy. 20x.

Figure 5.27 shows a feline fibrosarcoma biopsy. This 13-year-old neutered male Domestic Medium Hair cat had a previous necrotic mass removed from this same area 6 months earlier. The current mass was multinodular/multifocal and poorly circumscribed, and it involved the subcutis and deeper skeletal muscle. The mass is comprised of intersecting short bundles or fascicles of moderately pleomorphic polygonal and plump spindloid cells that appear fibroblastic. There is moderate variation in nuclear size. The cells have streaming eosinophilic cytoplasm with indistinct cell borders. Mitotic figures were easily found in this cell population. The centers of the nodules were somewhat rarefied and less cellular, and ischemic necrosis was multifocal in the centers of some of the nodules. There was also chronic perivascular lymphocytic and plasma cellular inflammation along portions of the periphery of the lesion. Margins could not be accurately assessed; lobules and nodules extended multifocally into various margins of the multicentric lesion submitted. Feline soft tissue sarcomas can be spontaneous, viral in origin, and can arise in the site of previous vaccination or injection (considered likely in this case.) Viral sarcomas, which are usually seen in young cats, may be multiple, but the others are usually solitary. In any case, the cells of origin are probably primitive myofibroblasts. The tumors differentiate to various types of mesenchymal tissue, fibrosarcoma, osteosarcoma, etc. These tumors are slow to metastasize but are famous for local recurrence, even if they appear to have been completely resected. Therefore, complete resection with very careful follow-up is usually advised, preferably after consultation with oncology and surgical specialists.

Figure 5.28 shows a feline soft tissue sarcoma FNA. This aspirate from the trunk of a 9-year-old Domestic Medium Hair cat reveals clusters of pleomorphic cells with marked anisokaryosis, multiple nuclei, nuclear nesting, prominent multiple nucleoli, and poorly defined basophilic cytoplasm. The preliminary diagnosis is sarcoma. Biopsy confirmation is suggested.

Figure 5.29 shows a recurrent feline fibrosarcoma, left hip biopsy. This 6-year-old spayed female Domestic Shorthair cat had a recurrent mass removed from the incision site on the left hip where a fibrosarcoma had been removed 4 months earlier. The new mass was more anaplastic, and it involved fibrovascular tissue, subcutis, and skeletal muscle. The mass was now a multilobular spindle cell neoplasm. In viable areas the cells are organized in broad interlacing bundles. In some areas the cells are densely packed with little stroma; in others they are more widely spaced with intervening connective tissue. The cells have variably sized oval to elongated open-faced nuclei with one or more prominent nucleoli. Mitoses were numerous in some areas. Cytoplasm is generally eosinophilic to vacuolated and streaming. There was chronic perivascular and nodular lymphocytic inflammation within the stroma of the mass in some areas and along portions of the periphery. Margins were clean but variable, and as narrow as 0.2 mm. Prognosis for long-term survival was considered guarded because this size margin is not considered adequate for this tumor type. Additional therapy is likely necessary for best prognosis, and consultation with a specialist is suggested.

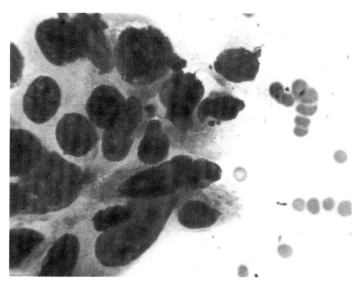

Figure 5.28 Feline soft tissue sarcoma FNA. 50x.

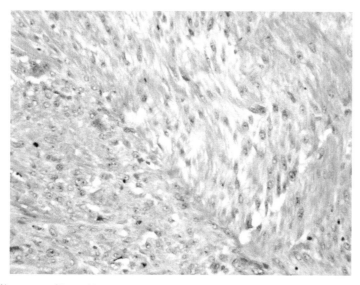

Figure 5.29 Recurrent feline fibrosarcoma biopsy. 20x.

Canine cutaneous lymphoma

Figure 5.30 shows a clinical presentation of canine cutaneous lymphoma on the skin of the right and left trunk.

Figure 5.31 shows a cutaneous lymphoma FNA. Aspirate of multifocal cutaneous masses, similar to those shown in Figure 5.30, can yield sheets of medium to large lymphocytes that are homogeneously larger than the few neutrophils present. This monomorphic population is typical of a neoplastic infiltrate when in the skin, as there is no significant resident population of lymphocytes in normal skin. This can be difficult to differentiate cytologically from histiocytoma, but histiocytoma generally is not multifocal and persistent.

Figure 5.32 shows a canine epitheliotrophic cutaneous malignant T-cell lymphoma, skin of trunk biopsy. A 14-year-old neutered male Maltese was presented with a month-long history of erythroderma progressing to scale and then to crusts with pruritus. There was no improvement with multiple antibiotics or antipruritic therapy. He also has depigmentation of the lips, muzzle, and periocular region. Cytology revealed lymphocytes. The skin biopsies were from the right and left trunk. No primary etiologic agents were recognized, and potential acantholytic cells were rare in crusts. The cells expanding the superficial dermis and forming coalescing festoons around pilosebaceous units are slightly enlarged somewhat pleomorphic polygonal and round cells that appear lymphoid. These cells are mononuclear, and they have nuclei slightly larger than red blood cell size with a central nucleolus. Potential mitoses were rare. The cells

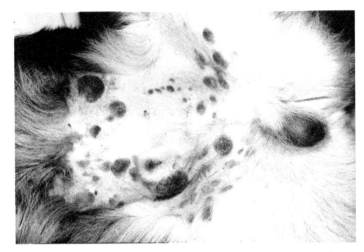

Figure 5.30 Clinical photograph of canine cutaneous lymphoma. (Courtesy of the College of Veterinary Medicine, University of Florida, Gainesville, FL.)

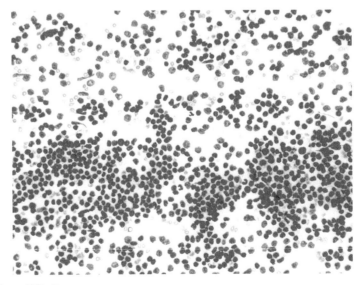

Figure 5.31 Cutaneous lymphoma FNA. 10x.

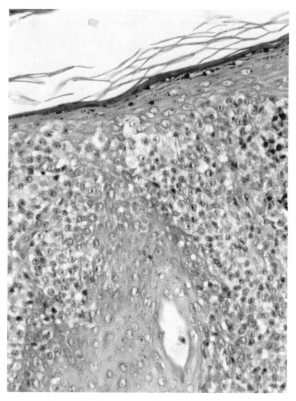

Figure 5.32 Canine epitheliotropic cutaneous malignant T-cell lymphoma biopsy. 20x.

multifocally infiltrate the epidermis and adnexal linings, sometimes forming recognizable Pautrier's microabscesses. This skin disease is also called mycosis fungoides. Secondary superficial pyoderma is a common complication. In canines this is usually a T-cell lymphoma. The lesions are multicentric, affecting skin and mucous membranes. They slowly progress from inflammatory foci, to thickened plaques, to actual tumor nodules. Lymph nodes and the peripheral blood can eventually become involved.

Mast cell tumor

Figure 5.33 shows a cutaneous mast cell tumor FNA. Aspiration of skin masses in the canine and feline can yield clusters of variably granulated mast cells, often with eosinophils and sometimes with stromal debris. One or two mast cells can elicit suspicion of a tumor but groups of mast cells usually indicate neoplasia.

Figure 5.34 shows a feline cutaneous mast cell tumor, left thorax, biopsy. An 8-year-old spayed female Domestic Shorthair cat was presented with two dermal masses on the left thorax. They were similar and caused by coalescent aggregates of slightly enlarged, poorly granular mast cells. There is little variation in cell and nuclear size, and mitoses were not seen. Margins were clean. The cells are still fairly well-differentiated with a low mitotic rate, but behavior of mast cell tumors is unpredictable in cats. These tumors may be multicentric, and they are capable of metastasis via lymphatics. These tumors are very often benign in behavior, even if they are cytologically pleomorphic and even if they are multiple.

Figure 5.35 shows a biopsy of a canine poorly granular high-grade mast cell tumor, subcutis of the right hip. A 10-year-old spayed female mixed breed canine was presented with a 10-cm-diameter soft tissue mass on the right hip that was resected and submitted for histopathology. The specimen is adipose and fibrovascular tissue with a diffusing infiltrate of round cells with moderate variation in cell and nuclear size. Cytoplasmic borders are distinct. MI = 8/10 HPF, and some cells have more than one nucleus. The mitotic rate is nonuniform. Varied numbers of eosinophils accompany the neoplastic cells. Giemsa stain reveals cytoplasmic metachromatic granules in the neoplastic cells, confirming that this is a rather poorly granular moderately pleomorphic mast cell tumor with an elevated mitotic rate, consistent with grade 3/high grade. Behavior of both low- and high-grade canine mast cell tumors is somewhat unpredictable. They are all capable of local recurrence, multicentric appearance, and metastasis via lymphatics. They are also likely to recur if not

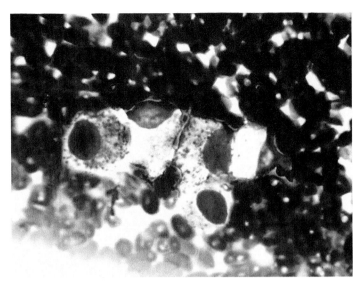

Figure 5.33 Cutaneous mast cell tumor FNA. 50x.

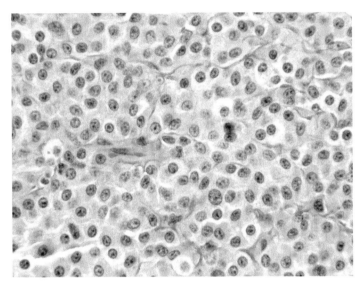

Figure 5.34 Feline cutaneous mast cell tumor biopsy. 40x.

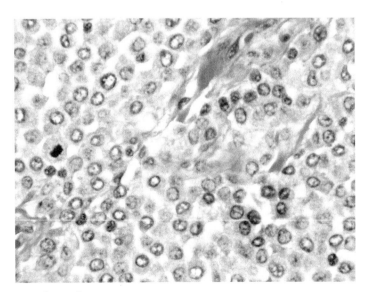

Figure 5.35 Canine cutaneous mast cell tumor biopsy. 40x.

completely and rather widely resected. Normal tissue margins of 2 cm laterally and one fascial plane deep are generally recommended but may not be possible depending on the location. Consultation with a specialist is recommended for the most current surgical recommendation and treatment options.

Canine histiocytoma

Figure 5.36 shows a canine histiocytoma FNA. Aspirate of a hairless, dome-shaped mass on the shoulder of a 1-year-old male Bulldog yielded many round cells with clear cytoplasm and round to reniform nuclei. The pale cytoplasm is clearly delineated when seen against a high protein background and is a hallmark of this generally benign tumor.

Figure 5.37 shows a biopsy of a canine histiocytoma. This 1-year-old spayed female mixed breed dog presented with an ulcerated, hairless, dome-shaped mass on the skin. Biopsy revealed medium-sized round to reniform cells that formed widely spaced radiating chains of cells in the subepidermis and occasionally infiltrated the epidermis. This occasional epitheliotrophism can mimic cutaneous lymphoma. Also, poorly granular mast cell tumor can sometimes look like histiocytoma with routine hematoxalin and eosin (H&E) stain. If the lesion appears of questionable etiology, Giemsa stain may be applied to this tissue as a special stain to exclude mast cell tumor, and immunohistochemistry can be performed to exclude lymphoid neoplasia.

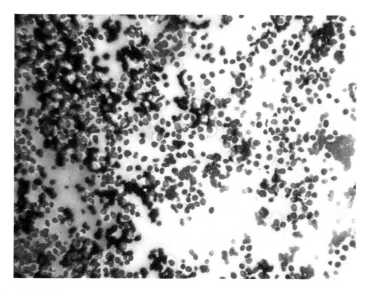

Figure 5.36   Canine histiocytoma FNA. 10x.

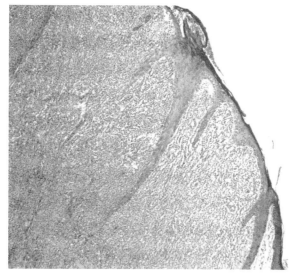

Figure 5.37   Canine histiocytoma biopsy. 10x.

Histiocytosis

Figure 5.38 shows feline histiocytosis FNA. Aspirate of a mass from a patient presenting with multifocal raised intradermal lesions may yield clusters of histiocytic cells that are morphologically similar to macrophages. These cells might contain phagocytosed debris. Differentials include granuloma or pyogranuloma formation, reactive histiocytosis, or neoplastic histiocytosis. A more aggressive disease such as histiocytic sarcoma can be considered if there is excessive nuclear pleomorphism or if internal organs are involved. Biopsy with routine H&E, as well as immunohistochemistry, may be necessary to identify the cell type, disease process, and prognosis.

Figure 5.39 shows a biopsy of a canine cutaneous histiocytosis, skin plaque on ventral thorax. Punch biopsies from erythematous plaques on the ventrum of a 5-year-old neutered male Doberman Pinscher were submitted. They revealed a mixed but mostly histiocytic infiltrate that was periadnexal, perivascular, multinodular, and diffusing, involving the dermis and superficial subcutis. The infiltrates were poorly circumscribed. They are comprised of fairly large polygonal cells that appear histiocytic. These cells are accompanied by individual neutrophils, lymphocytes, and plasma cells. Near the deep borders are loose aggregates of lymphocytes and plasma cells. Most of the histiocytic cells are mononuclear. Scattered cells have more than one nucleus. Mitotic figures were found in this cell population, but the

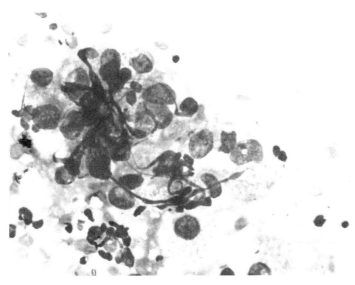

Figure 5.38 Feline histiocytosis FNA. 40x.

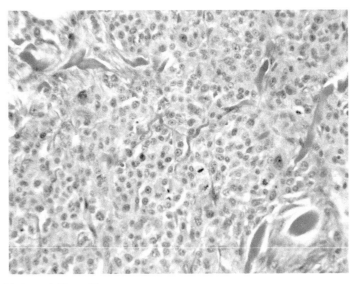

Figure 5.39 Canine cutaneous histiocytosis biopsy. 20x.

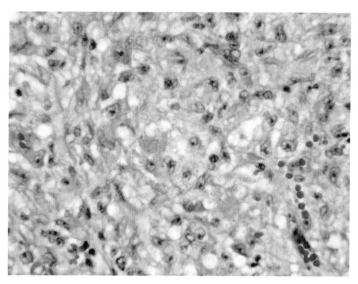

Figure 5.40 Presumptive feline cutaneous progressive histiocytosis biopsy. 40x.

mitotic rate was non-uniform. Margins of the plaques could not be assessed. The primary histologic differential was reactive histiocytosis (cutaneous histiocytosis if only the skin is involved). Histiocytosis can become systemic, involving lymph nodes and internal organs.

Figure 5.40 shows a biopsy of a presumptive feline cutaneous progressive histiocytosis of the tail. A 16-year-old spayed female Domestic Shorthair cat was presented for a mass on the tail. The surface was ulcerated, exudative, and crusted, and the mass was multinodular. It is comprised of histiocytic cells with a few neutrophils, individual eosinophils, and scattered perivascular and small nodular aggregates of lymphocytes and plasma cells. The cells were infiltrating the dermis and subcutis. Histiocytic infiltrates were also noted in the dermis peripheral to the primary mass, associated with the large lobules of hepatoid sebaceous glands in this location. No primary etiologic agents were seen. Margins were clean. This lesion appears inflammatory and reactive, and progressive feline histiocytosis was the primary histologic differential. However, those lesions are usually multicentric, and no other lesions were reported. It is unknown whether or not this patient had ever received an injection in the skin of the tail at the site of the lesion, as has been suggested for feline rabies vaccinations, and no follow-up information was available.

Dorsal tail head masses

Pilomatricoma

Figure 5.41 shows feline pilomatricoma FNA. Aspirate of a circumscribed, freely movable mass in the skin of the dorsal back may yield scattered small basaloid cells and melanin-laden macrophages in a background of cellular debris and melanin. It may not be possible to differentiate this from a melanoma without biopsy.

Figure 5.42 shows a feline pilomatricoma biopsy. This mass is from the right shoulder of a 7-year-old spayed female Domestic Shorthair cat. This tumor type arises from hair matrix cells. The mass was a multilobular/multinodular epithelial neoplasm comprised mostly of multilayered basaloid cells that line cysts containing eosinophilic granular debris, amorphous keratin, and clumps of degenerating pigmented epithelial cells. Scattered pigmented cells were noted throughout the walls of many of the cysts, as well. There were only hints at squamous differentiation of the basaloid cells along portions of the inner linings of the cysts of varied size. Stromal invasion and intra-lymphatic spread were not seen in the periphery, but there was some chronic lymphocytic and plasma cellular inflammation around the periphery, especially along the base. Margins were clean. These tumors are usually benign and solitary.

Melanoma

Figure 5.43 shows a canine well-differentiated dermal melanoma FNA. Aspiration of a dark skin mass on the rump of an adult neutered male Schnauzer revealed epithelioid cells with dense cytoplasmic melanin granules in a background of cellular debris and melanin. This is cytologically compatible with a melanoma. Biopsy is necessary to determine the mitotic rate for prognosis.

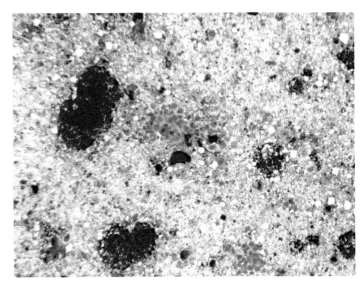

Figure 5.41 Feline pilomatricoma FNA. 10x.

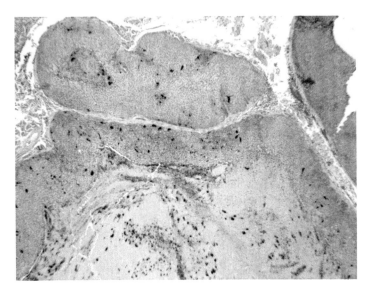

Figure 5.42 Feline pilomatricoma biopsy. 4x.

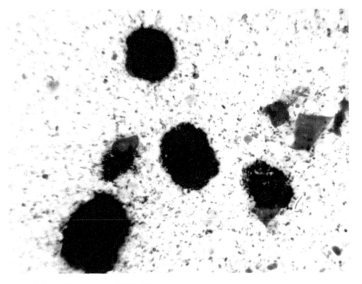

Figure 5.43 Canine well-differentiated dermal melanoma FNA. 50x.

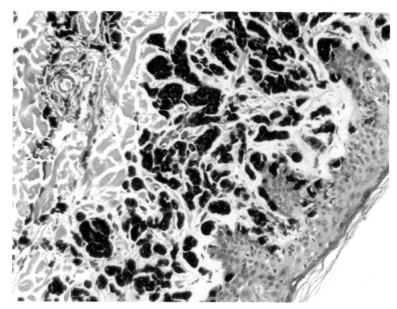

Figure 5.44 Canine well-differentiated dermal melanoma biopsy. 10x.

Figure 5.44 shows a biopsy of a canine well-differentiated dermal melanoma. A 7-year-old neutered male Mastiff presented with a pigmented skin mass on the flank. Biopsy revealed skin with an epidermal/subepidermal interface and subepidermal proliferation of nests of deeply pigmented melanocytes. Mitotic figures are not seen, and the lesion is considered well-differentiated and potentially not aggressive.

Figure 5.45 shows a canine poorly differentiated melanoma FNA. Aspirate of a mass on the back of a 12-year-old mixed breed dog revealed clusters of pleomorphic spindloid to epithelioid, occasionally multinucleate, cells with multiple small nucleoli and scant cytoplasmic melanin. The preliminary diagnosis is poorly melanotic melanoma, which is cytologically poorly differentiated and likely aggressive. Biopsy is recommended to evaluate the mitotic rate and give prognosis.

Figure 5.46 shows a canine malignant dermal melanoma, right trunk biopsy. A 10-year-old spayed female mixed breed canine was presented with a hemorrhagic skin mass on the right trunk. The mass was covered by stratified squamous epithelium, which varied in thickness from acanthotic to attenuated. At the edges of the mass, junctional activity was recognized as aggregates of enlarged melanocytic cells dropping off the basement membrane of the epidermis into the dermis. The mass is comprised of pleomorphic medium to fairly large polygonal and round cells with a prominent central nucleolus and varying amounts of cytoplasm. Many cells are unpigmented, but cells of varied pigmentation are present. Scattered individual heavily pigmented melanophages are also present. MI = 12/ HPF, but distribution of mitotic figures varied considerably. Margins were clean. Canine dermal melanomas are often multiple. They can be found anywhere on the skin, and skin of the trunk is a relatively common site. They are usually benign in behavior, at least for extended periods of time, but they can undergo malignant transformation, as in this case. Malignant varieties may recur even if completely resected, and they can eventually metastasize via lymphatics.

Masses on the dorsum of the tail head are occasionally submitted. The presence of active glands at this site may be related to residual scent-marking apparatus. Sebaceous, apocrine, and perianal gland structures are typically seen at this site.

Sebaceous adenoma

Figure 5.47 shows a feline sebaceous gland proliferation, tail head, FNA. This aspirate from a skin mass on an adult male Domestic Shorthair cat reveals clusters of well-differentiated sebaceous gland epithelium. Preliminary diagnosis is sebaceous gland proliferation, and biopsy is recommended to determine the type. Sebaceous glands of the skin on the tail head can sometimes proliferate, possibly in response to androgenic adrenal hormones.

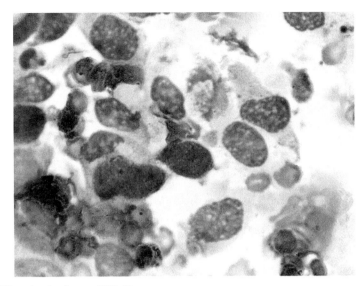

Figure 5.45 Canine poorly differentiated melanoma FNA. 50x.

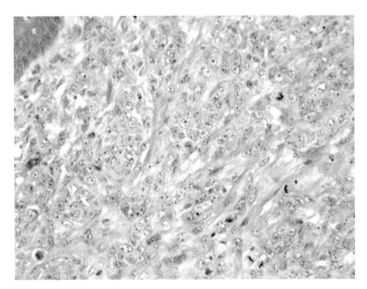

Figure 5.46 Canine malignant dermal melanoma biopsy. 20x.

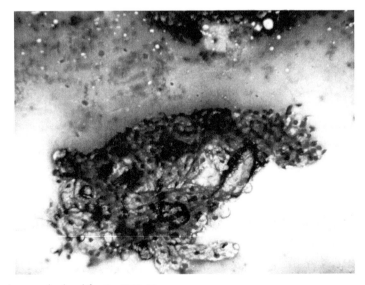

Figure 5.47 Feline tail head sebaceous gland proliferation FNA. 10x.

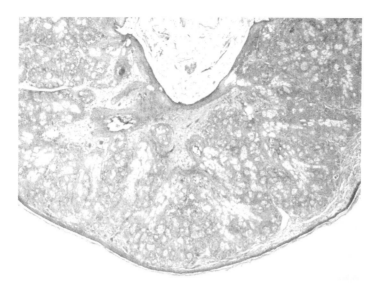

Figure 5.48 Canine tail head sebaceous gland adenoma biopsy. 10x.

Figure 5.48 shows a biopsy of a canine tail head sebaceous gland adenoma. An 11-year-old spayed female Maltese dog presented with a dorsal tail head mass. Biopsy revealed a well-differentiated but somewhat disorganized proliferation of sebaceous glands around a dilated keratin-filled cystic duct.

Perianal gland adenoma

Figure 5.49 shows a canine perianal gland adenoma FNA. Aspirate of a dorsal tail head mass on an adult spayed female mixed breed dog revealed clusters of hepatoid epithelial cells with small nuclei in abundant vaguely granular eosinophilic cytoplasm. Ectopic proliferation of perianal gland tissue may cause masses on the dorsal tail head of male and female dogs.

Figure 5.50 shows a biopsy of a canine perianal gland adenoma. A 13-year-old male Poodle dog presented with a dorsal tail head mass. Biopsy revealed clusters of hepatoid cells with small nuclei in abundant eosinophilic cytoplasm, arranged in lobules lined by a thin layer of basaloid reserve cells. This tumor is hormone responsive, and complete excision with castration can be curative.

Ventral trunk vascular lesions of the skin and subcutis

Cutaneous vascular lesions tend to present as discolored, bloody, or bruised lesions. If there is no history of trauma and no clinical evidence of coagulopathy or thrombocytopenia, biopsy is warranted.

Figure 5.51 shows a clinical presentation of canine cutaneous hemangiosarcoma with extensive extravasation. This can be mistaken for traumatic injury so a thorough history is warranted.

Hemangioma

Figure 5.52 shows a canine hemangioma FNA. Aspiration of a dark-colored raised skin mass on the ventral abdomen of an aged Italian Greyhound dog yielded peripheral blood. The presence of platelets suggests acute hemorrhage, which can also be seen with acute hematoma, coagulopathy, or inadvertent venipuncture.

Figure 5.53 shows a canine subcutaneous hemangioma, left abdomen biopsy. A mass of large blood-filled spaces lined by flattened well-differentiated endothelial cells and separated by somewhat hyalinized fibrous connective tissue trabeculae was fairly well circumscribed but unencapsulated. Individual mast cells and small aggregates of lymphocytes and plasma cells were scattered in the stroma. Margins on the sections were clean. This vascular tumor appears bland and benign histologically. Such tumors may be multiple and can become quite numerous in the skin. Surgical excision is the treatment of choice.

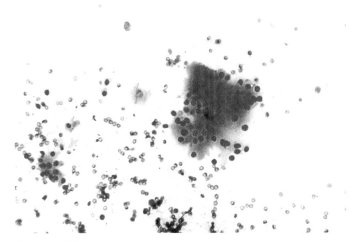

Figure 5.49 Canine perianal gland adenoma FNA. 10x.

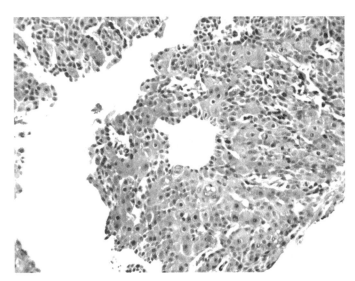

Figure 5.50 Canine perianal gland adenoma biopsy. 10x.

Hemangiosarcoma

Figure 5.54 shows a canine hemangiosarcoma FNA. Aspiration of a diffuse, ulcerated, and bleeding superficial mass on the ventral abdomen of a 10-year-old female Bulldog yielded blood with platelet clumps, many neutrophils, and a giant and atypical mitotic figure (arrow). The presence of pleomorphic epithelioid to spindloid cells or, in this case, a giant and atypical mitotic figure, suggests sarcomatous neoplasia. Biopsy is necessary for definitive diagnosis of vascular tumors.

Figure 5.55 shows a canine hemangiosarcoma, ventral abdomen biopsy. A 7-year-old spayed female Greyhound had an enlarging mass on the abdomen that became hemorrhagic. The surface was focally ulcerated. The intact stratified squamous epidermis was acanthotic. The poorly circumscribed mass is comprised of pleomorphic enlarged vascular endothelial cells with large nuclei, a prominent nucleolus, and scant cytoplasm. The cells sometimes have more than one nucleus. They line anastomosing capillary and more cavernous blood-filled spaces. Mitotic figures were found in this cell population. There was chronic inflammation peripheral to the mass, with some inflammation in the stroma. Margins were clean but multifocally narrow. This mass is a cutaneous hemangiosarcoma, which was already involving the superficial subcutis (T2). Canine vascular endothelial neoplasms are frequently multiple and sometimes numerous. They tend to develop in areas of chronic actinic damage, so the poorly haired skin of the ventrum is a common site. There is an increased incidence in this breed. Regularly scheduled skin checks were recommended for this patient. Also, the owner was advised that the patient should be protected from the sun from now on (direct sunlight from sunbathing and reflected light from walking on light cement or sandy surfaces).

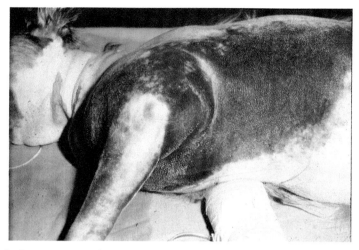

Figure 5.51 Clinical photograph of canine cutaneous hemangiosarcoma with extensive extravasation. (Courtesy of the College of Veterinary Medicine, University of Florida, Gainesville, FL.)

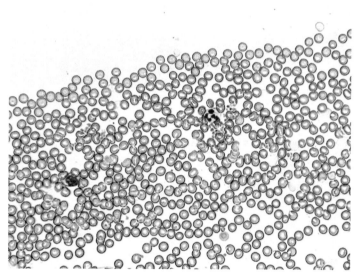

Figure 5.52 Canine hemangioma FNA. 10x.

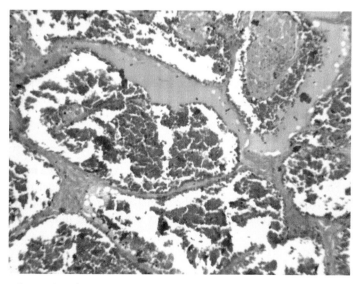

Figure 5.53 Canine subcutaneous hemangioma biopsy. 10x.

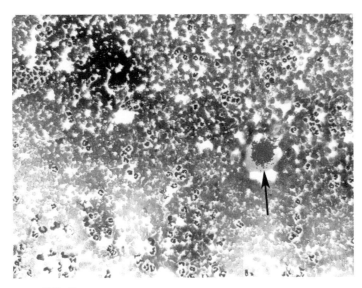

Figure 5.54 Canine hemangiosarcoma FNA. 50x.

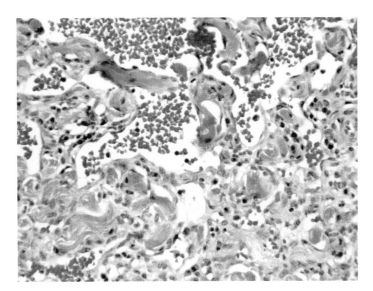

Figure 5.55 Canine hemangiosarcoma biopsy. 20x.

Mass lesions of the mammary gland

Mammary gland neoplasia is frequent in dogs and occasional in cats. Dogs exhibit a wide range of tumor types from benign to malignant. Cat tumors are less varied in behavior, and all masses are suspected of aggressive potential except in the case of intact females that may be undergoing cyclical hormonal stimulation.

Fibroepithelial hyperplasia

Figure 5.56 shows a feline mammary fibroepithelial hyperplasia FNA. An aspirate of a mammary mass from a 1-year-old intact female Domestic Shorthair cat revealed spindle cells with small oblong nuclei and a few scattered epithelial cells with small nuclei. This is a hyperplastic response by the epithelial and myoepithelial layers of the mammary gland to hormonal stimulation such as pseudopregnancy. It can affect one gland or multiple glands. It is benign and will regress with decreased hormone levels.

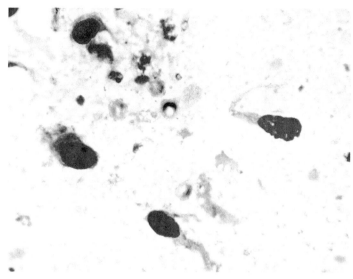

Figure 5.56 Feline mammary fibroepithelial hyperplasia FNA. 50x.

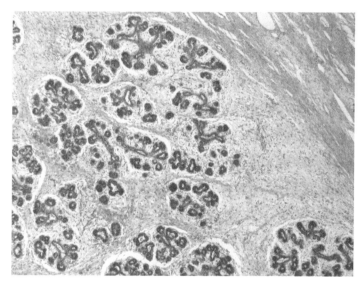

Figure 5.57 Canine mammary fibroepithelial hyperplasia biopsy. 10x.

Figure 5.57 shows a canine mammary fibroepithelial hyperplasia biopsy. This biopsy from the mammary gland of an 8-year-old female Labrador Retriever dog shows well-defined lobules of plump tubuloalveolar epithelium surrounded by proliferating slender spindle cells. This proliferation of epithelial and stromal cells forms a nodule within the normal fibrovascular stroma.

Mammary gland adenoma

Figure 5.58 shows a mammary gland well-differentiated proliferation FNA. An aspirate of a mammary mass on an 8-year-old spayed female Dachshund revealed clusters of small epithelial cells with small, dense, round nuclei. There is a vague acinar appearance to some clusters of cells. This well-differentiated proliferation of mammary gland epithelium is compatible with adenoma.

Figure 5.59 shows a canine mammary tubular adenoma biopsy. This mammary mass is from a 10-year-old spayed female Labrador Retriever. The mass was multilobular and partially intraductal. It is comprised of somewhat pleomorphic epithelial cells that form acini and tubules. Some tubules contain papillary proliferations of branching glands.

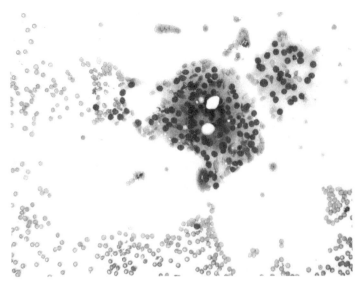

Figure 5.58 Canine mammary gland adenoma FNA. 10x.

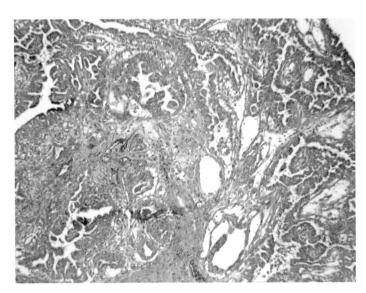

Figure 5.59 Canine mammary tubular adenoma biopsy. 4x.

Stromal invasion and intralymphatic spread were not recognized around the periphery. The surrounding mammary tissue was relatively inactive. Margins on the sections were clean. Expected behavior is as described above. Resection should be curative, but mammary tumors are often multiple in this species.

Complex adenoma

Figure 5.60 shows a canine mammary complex adenoma FNA. Aspiration of a mammary mass on a 5-year-old Spitz dog revealed a proliferation of plump epithelial cells with mild to moderate anisokaryosis (arrow), occasional prominent nucleoli, and variably basophilic cytoplasm with occasional spindle cells (arrowhead) in a background of blood. The presence of both epithelioid and spindloid cells implies a complex tumor, but biopsy is necessary for definitive diagnosis.

Figure 5.61 shows a canine complex mammary adenoma biopsy. This mammary mass is from a 9-year-old spayed female English Springer Spaniel. The mass was multilobular and multinodular, and sometimes intraductal. There is an epithelial and a myoepithelial or mesenchymal component. The epithelial component is somewhat pleomorphic and forms ductules, acini, and trabecular cords, and there are also papillary proliferations into the lumina of dilated ducts in some areas. The myoepithelial element is less cellular, and the cells are more spindloid. Ground substance is

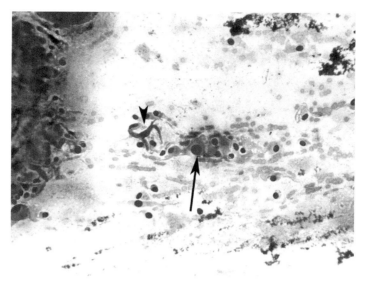

Figure 5.60 Canine mammary complex adenoma FNA. 4x.

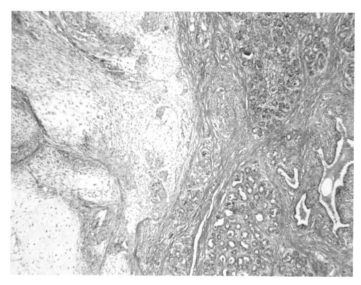

Figure 5.61 Canine complex mammary adenoma biopsy. 4x.

sometimes hyalinized but mostly faintly mucinous in the area pictured. There was no evidence of stromal invasion or intralymphatic spread around the peripheral of the lobules and nodules. The surrounding mammary tissue was somewhat hyperplastic with mild adenomatous hyperplasia. Margins of this neoplastic mass were clean. Over 50% of the time mammary tumors are benign in canines, but they are frequently multiple. These tumors can undergo malignant transformation. The epithelial element is most often involved, becoming malignant and eventually metastasizing via lymphatics to draining lymph nodes, then elsewhere, if the neoplasm is very chronic. The sparing effect of ovariectomy only occurs if the animal was spayed prior to the second estrus.

Mixed mammary tumor

Figure 5.62 shows a canine mammary mixed mammary tumor FNA. There is a proliferation of plump epithelial cells with mild to moderate anisokaryosis, occasional prominent nucleoli, and variably basophilic cytoplasm with occasional spindle cells in a background of blood and clusters of eosinophilic to lightly basophilic material (arrows) suggestive of osteoid or cartilage matrix. The presence of matrix typical of bone or cartilage suggests a mixed mammary tumor. Biopsy is necessary for definitive diagnosis.

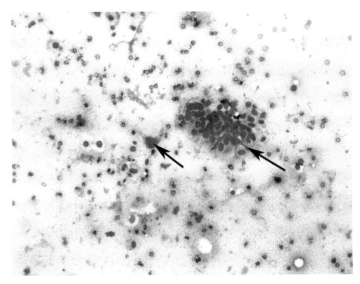

Figure 5.62 Canine mammary mixed mammary tumor FNA. 40x.

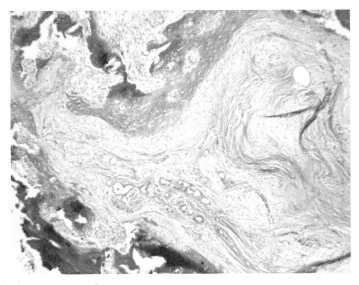

Figure 5.63 Canine benign mixed mammary tumor biopsy. 4x.

Figure 5.63 shows a canine benign mixed mammary tumor with bony metaplasia biopsy. This mammary mass is from an 11-year-old spayed female Chinese Crested Dog. The mass was multilobular and sometimes intraductal with an epithelial and a myoepithelial or mesenchymal component. The epithelial component was multifocally cystic. Within the mesenchymal component were hints at cartilaginous differentiation and also multifocal formation of well-differentiated bone. There was no evidence of stromal invasion or intralymphatic spread around the periphery. The associated mammary tissue appeared to be inactive. Margins of the mass were clean, so resection was expected to be curative for this individual tumor.

Mammary carcinoma

Figure 5.64 shows a canine mammary carcinoma FNA. Aspiration of a mammary mass on a 9-year-old spayed female Chihuahua dog reveals clusters of cells with large nuclei, moderate anisokaryosis, and basophilic cytoplasm. A preliminary diagnosis of carcinoma is suggested if there are numerous clusters of this type of cell or if there are cells with marked anisokaryosis, as canine mammary tumors overall have only a moderate probability of aggressive behavior.

Figure 5.65 shows a canine scirrhous mammary tubular adenocarcinoma with intralymphatic embolization biopsy. A subcutaneous mass was submitted from the ventral abdomen of an 8-year-old spayed female mixed breed canine.

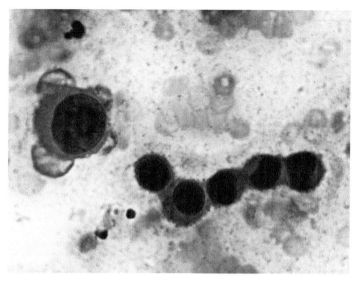

Figure 5.64 Canine mammary carcinoma FNA. 40x.

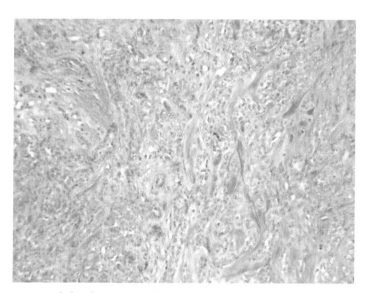

Figure 5.65 Canine scirrhous mammary tubular adenocarcinoma biopsy. 10x.

The poorly circumscribed infiltrative mass suffered multifocal ischemic necrosis with some replacement fibrosis. It is comprised of moderately pleomorphic polygonal and round cells with moderate variation in cell and nuclear size. These cells form solid aggregates. They also line acini and branching tubules in one to multiple layers. The stroma is dense, intensely eosinophilic, and hyalinized. There is chronic perivascular and nodular lymphocytic inflammation all along the periphery, especially in areas of stromal invasion by the neoplasm. There was at least one intralymphatic embolus (not shown). Margins could not be assessed with confidence because the specimen was submitted in two partial pieces. Metastasis to draining lymph nodes and then to more distant sites was expected.

Figure 5.66 shows a feline mammary carcinoma FNA. Aspiration of a mass on a 6-year-old spayed female Birman cat reveals scattered clusters of pleomorphic epithelial cells with a few large epithelial cells exhibiting marked aniso-karyosis, large nucleoli, and basophilic cytoplasm. Finding even a few of these large cells is suggestive of carcinoma in a cat because feline mammary tumors overall have a high probability of aggressive behavior.

Figure 5.67 shows a feline mammary carcinoma, ventral thorax biopsy. A 13-year-old spayed female Domestic Shorthair cat had a mass on the ventral thorax. The mass was actually multicentric. It has a fairly dense fibrous connective tissue stroma, and it is composed of medium to large polygonal epithelial cells with moderate variation in cell and

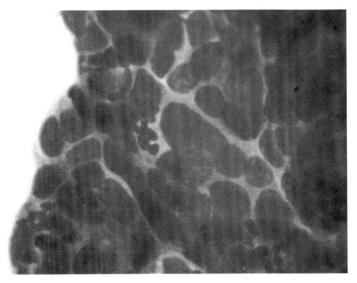

Figure 5.66 Feline mammary carcinoma FNA. 50x.

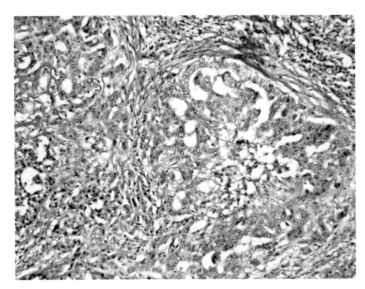

Figure 5.67 Feline mammary carcinoma biopsy. 10x.

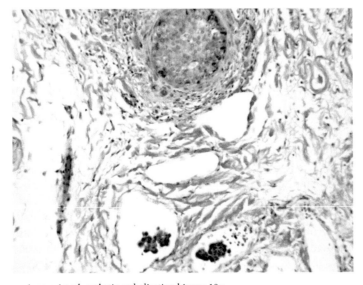

Figure 5.68 Canine mammary carcinoma, intralymphatic embolization biopsy. 10x.

nuclear size, mostly very large nuclei with a large single nucleolus, and a moderate amount of eosinophilic cytoplasm. These cells form acini, tubules, and trabecular cords. Mitoses were seen in this cell population at a rate of 0–4/HPF, and some cells had more than one nucleus. Abnormal mitotic spindles were present. There were small nodules peripheral to the primary mass in one area that were suspected to be within lymphatics. The neoplasm extended into the subcutaneous margin in this area, and the masses appeared partially peeled out in other areas. Feline mammary tumors are malignant in behavior much of the time. They are also often multicentric. They can recur rather quickly even if completely resected, they readily metastasize to draining lymph nodes, and they also spread to other sites, especially the lungs. Therefore, the prognosis for long-term survival was considered poor in this case. Consultation with a specialist prior to surgery is recommended for current treatment options due to the high probability of recurrence of this tumor type.

Figure 5.68 shows a canine mammary carcinoma, intralymphatic embolization biopsy. A 9-year-old spayed female Doberman cross canine had a large subcutaneous inguinal mass diagnosed as a solid and cystic adenocarcinoma. Intralymphatic emboli were disseminating in all directions around the primary mass. A group of small tumor nodules, some within lymphatics, extended just to the deep margin of the specimen. Recurrence and metastasis to regional lymph nodes and then to more distant sites was predicted.

Additional reading

Mass lesions of the dorsal trunk

Raskin RE. Skin and Subcutaneous Tissues. In Canine and Feline Cytology; A Color Atlas and Interpretation Guide. 3rd ed. Raskin and Meyer. 2016. Elsevier. St. Louis. 34–90.

Fisher DJ. Cutaneous and Subcutaneous Lesions. In Cowell and Tyler's Diagnostic Cytology and Hematology of the Dog and Cat. 4th ed. Valenciano and Cowell. 2014. 80–109.

Hauck ML. Tumors of the Skin and Subcutaneous Tissues. In In Small Animal Clinical Oncology, 5th ed. Withrow and MacEwen. 2013. Elsevier. St. Louis. 305–320.

Mauldin EA, Peters-Kennedy J. Integumentary System. In Jubb, Kennedy and Palmer's Pathology of Domestic Animals. Vol 1. 6th ed. M. Grant Maxie, Editor. Elsevier. St Louis. 2016. 509–736.

Calcinosis cutis

Gross TL, Ihrke PJ, Walder EJ, Affolter VK. Degenerative, dysplastic and depositional diseases of dermal connective tissue. In Skin Diseases of the Dog and Cat; Clinical and Histopathologic Diagnosis. 2nd ed. 2005. Blackwell Publishing. Oxford. 373–403.

Follicular cyst
Cystic adnexal tumors—tricoepithelioma, keratoachanthoma

de Lorimier LP. Hair Follicle Tumors. In Blackwell's Five-Minute Veterinary Consult: Canine and Feline. 5th ed. Tilley LP and Smith FWK, Jr. 2011. John Wiley & Sons, Inc. West Sussex, UK. 528.

Gross TL, Ihrke PJ, Walder EJ, and Affolter VK. Follicular Tumors. In Skin Diseases of the Dog and Cat; Clinical and Histopathologic Diagnosis. 2nd ed. 2005. Blackwell Publishing. Oxford. 604–640.

Apocrine adenoma
Apocrine and sebaceous carcinoma

de Lorimier LP. Adenocarcinoma, Skin (Sweat Gland, Sebaceous). In Blackwell's Five-Minute Veterinary Consult: Canine and Feline. 5th ed. Tilley LP and Smith FWK, Jr. 2011. John Wiley & Sons, Inc. West Sussex, UK. 31.

Gross TL, Ihrke PJ, Walder EJ, Affolter VK. Sweat gland Tumors. In Skin Diseases of the Dog and Cat; Clinical and Histopathologic Diagnosis. 2nd ed. 2005. Blackwell Publishing. Oxford. 665–694.

Lipoma

Gross TL, Ihrke PJ, Walder EJ, Affolter VK. Lipocytic Tumors. In Skin Diseases of the Dog and Cat; Clinical and Histopathologic Diagnosis. 2nd ed. 2005. Blackwell Publishing. Oxford. 766–777.

Mutsaers AJ. Lipoma. In Blackwell's Five-Minute Veterinary Consult: Canine and Feline. 5th ed. Tilley LP and Smith FWK, Jr. 2011. John Wiley & Sons, Inc. West Sussex, UK. 752.

Canine well-differentiated spindle cell proliferation

Gross TL, Ihrke PJ, Walder EJ, Affolter VK. Diseases of the Panniculus. In Skin Diseases of the Dog and Cat; Clinical and Histopathologic Diagnosis. 2nd ed. 2005. Blackwell Publishing. Oxford. 538–558.

Kuntz CA, Dernell WS, Powers BE, et al. JAVMA. 1997. 211:1147–1151.

Canine spindle cell tumor, mid grade
Canine spindle cell tumor, high grade
Feline spindle cell tumor

Gross TL, Ihrke PJ, Walder EJ, Affolter VK. Fibrous Tumors. In Skin Diseases of the Dog and Cat; Clinical and Histopathologic Diagnosis. 2nd ed. 2005. Blackwell Publishing. Oxford. 710–734.

Gross TL, Ihrke PJ, Walder EJ, Affolter VK. Perivascular Tumors. In Skin Diseases of the Dog and Cat; Clinical and Histopathologic Diagnosis. 2nd ed. 2005. Blackwell Publishing. Oxford. 759–765.

Gross TL, Ihrke PJ, Walder EJ, and Affolter VK. Smooth Muscle and Skeletal Muscle Tumors. In Skin Diseases of the Dog and Cat; Clinical and Histopathologic Diagnosis. 2nd ed. 2005. Blackwell Publishing. Oxford. 778–785.

Gross TL, Ihrke PJ, Walder EJ, Affolter VK. Neural and Perineural Tumors. In Skin Diseases of the Dog and Cat; Clinical and Histopathologic Diagnosis. 2nd ed. 2005. Blackwell Publishing. Oxford. 786–796.

Gross TL, Ihrke PJ, Walder EJ, and Affolter VK. Other MesenchymalTumors. In Skin Diseases of the Dog and Cat; Clinical and Histopathologic Diagnosis. 2nd ed. 2005. Blackwell Publishing. Oxford. 797–812.

Kuntz CA, Dernell WS, Powers BE, et al. JAVMA. 1997. 211:1147–1151.

Liptak JM, Forrest LJ. Soft Tissue Sarcomas. In Small Animal Clinical Oncology, 5th ed. Withrow and MacEwen. 2013. Elsevier. St. Louis. 356–380.

Morrison WB. Vaccine-Associated Sarcoma. In Blackwell's Five-Minute Veterinary Consult: Canine and Feline. 5th ed. Tilley LP and Smith FWK, Jr. 2011. John Wiley & Sons, Inc. West Sussex, UK. 1284–85.

Canine cutaneous lymphoma

Gross TL, Ihrke PJ, Walder EJ, Affolter VK. Lymphocytic Tumors. In Skin Diseases of the Dog and Cat; Clinical and Histopathologic Diagnosis. 2nd ed. 2005. Blackwell Publishing. Oxford. 866–893.

Torres S. Lymphoma, Cutaneous Epitheliotropic. In Blackwell's Five-Minute Veterinary Consult: Canine and Feline. 5th ed. Tilley LP and Smith FWK, Jr. 2011. John Wiley & Sons, Inc. West Sussex, UK. 780.

Mast cell tumor

Gross TL, Ihrke PJ, Walder EJ, Affolter VK. Mast Cell Tumors. In Skin Diseases of the Dog and Cat; Clinical and Histopathologic Diagnosis. 2nd ed. 2005. Blackwell Publishing. Oxford. 853–865.

London CA, Thamm DH. Mast Cell Tumors. In Small Animal Clinical Oncology, 5th ed. Withrow and MacEwen. 2013. Elsevier. St. Louis. 335–355.

Wilson-Robles HM. Mast Cell Tumors. In Blackwell's Five-Minute Veterinary Consult: Canine and Feline. 5th ed. Tilley LP and Smith FWK, Jr. 2011. John Wiley & Sons, Inc. West Sussex, UK. 795–796.

Canine histiocytoma
Histiocytosis

Clifford CA. Histiocytoma. In Blackwell's Five-Minute Veterinary Consult: Canine and Feline. 5th ed. Tilley LP and Smith FWK, Jr. 2011. John Wiley & Sons, Inc. West Sussex, UK. 585.

Clifford CA, Skorupski KA, Moore PF. Histiocytic Diseases. In Small Animal Clinical Oncology, 5th ed. Withrow and MacEwen. 2013. Elsevier. St. Louis. 706–715.

Gross TL, Ihrke PJ, Walder EJ, Affolter VK. Histiocytic Tumors. In Skin Diseases of the Dog and Cat; Clinical and Histopathologic Diagnosis. 2nd ed. 2005. Blackwell Publishing. Oxford. 837–852.

Hirako A, Sugiyama A, Sakurai M, et al. Cutaneous histiocytic sarcoma with E-cadherin expression in a Pembroke Welsh Corgi dog. 2015. JVDI 27:589–595.

Dorsal tail head masses

Hauck ML. Tumors of the Skin and Subcutaneous Tissues. In Small Animal Clinical Oncology, 5th ed. Withrow and MacEwen. 2013. Elsevier. St. Louis. 305–320.

Pilomatricoma

Gross TL, Ihrke PJ, Walder EJ, Affolter VK. Follicular Tumors. In Skin Diseases of the Dog and Cat; Clinical and Histopathologic Diagnosis. 2nd ed. 2005. Blackwell Publishing. Oxford. 604–640.

Melanoma

Bergman PJ, Kent MS, Farese JP. Melanoma. In In Small Animal Clinical Oncology, 5th ed. Withrow and MacEwen. 2013. Elsevier. St. Louis. 305–320.

Gross TL, Ihrke PJ, Walder EJ, Affolter VK. Melanocytic Tumors. In Skin Diseases of the Dog and Cat; Clinical and Histopathologic Diagnosis. 2nd ed. 2005. Blackwell Publishing. Oxford. 813–836.

Sebaceous adenoma
Perianal gland adenoma

Gross TL, Ihrke PJ, Walder EJ, and Affolter VK. Sebaceous Tumors. In Skin Diseases of the Dog and Cat; Clinical and Histopathologic Diagnosis. 2nd ed. 2005. Blackwell Publishing. Oxford. 641–664.

Turek MM, Withrow SJ. Perianal tumors. In Small Animal Clinical Oncology, 5th ed. Withrow and MacEwen. 2013. Elsevier. St. Louis. 423–431.

Ventral trunk vascular lesions of the skin and subcutis

Hemangioma
Hemangiosarcoma

Clifford C. Hemangiosarcoma, Skin. In Blackwell's Five-Minute Veterinary Consult: Canine and Feline. 5th ed. Tilley LP and Smith FWK, Jr. 2011. John Wiley & Sons, Inc. West Sussex, UK. 544.

Gross TL, Ihrke PJ, Walder EJ, Affolter VK. Vascular Tumors. In Skin Diseases of the Dog and Cat; Clinical and Histopathologic Diagnosis. 2nd ed. 2005. Blackwell Publishing. Oxford. 735–758.

Robinson WF, Robinson NA. Cardiovascular System. In Jubb, Kennedy and Palmer's Pathology of Domestic Animals. Vol 3. 6th ed. M. Grant Maxie, Editor. Elsevier. St Louis. 2016. 1–101.

Thamm DH. Hemangiosarcoma. In Small Animal Clinical Oncology, 5th ed. Withrow and MacEwen. 2013. Elsevier. St. Louis. 679–688.

Mass lesions of the mammary gland

Allison RW. Subcutaneous Glandular Tissue: Mammary, Salivary, Thyroid, and Parathyroid. In Cowell and Tyler's Diagnostic Cytology and Hematology of the Dog and Cat. 4th ed. Valenciano and Cowell. 110–130.

Schlafer DH, Foster RA. Female Genital System. In Jubb, Kennedy and Palmer's Pathology of Domestic Animals. Vol 3. 6th ed. M. Grant Maxie editor. Elsevier. St Louis. 2016. 358–464.

Sorenmo KU, Worley DR, Goldschmidt MH. Tumors of the Mammary Gland. In Small Animal Clinical Oncology, 5th ed. Withrow and MacEwen. 2013. Elsevier. St. Louis. 538–556.

Solano-Gallego L, Masserdotti C. Reproductive System. In Canine and Feline Cytology; A Color Atlas and Interpretation Guide. 3rd ed. Raskin and Meyer. 2016. Elsevier. St. Louis. 313–352.

Fibroepithelial hyperplasia

Root Kustritz MV. Mammary Gland Hyperplasia-Cats. In Blackwell's Five-Minute Veterinary Consult: Canine and Feline. 5th ed. Tilley LP and Smith FWK, Jr. 2011. John Wiley & Sons, Inc. West Sussex, UK. 786.

Mammary carcinoma

Morrison WB. Mammary Gland Tumors-Dogs. In Blackwell's Five-Minute Veterinary Consult: Canine and Feline. 5th ed. Tilley LP and Smith FWK, Jr. 2011. John Wiley & Sons, Inc. West Sussex, UK. 789–790.

Bailey DB. Mammary Gland Tumors-Cats. In Blackwell's Five-Minute Veterinary Consult: Canine and Feline. 5th ed. Tilley LP and Smith FWK, Jr. 2011. John Wiley & Sons, Inc. West Sussex, UK. 787–788.

Selected Lesions of the Thoracic Viscera

Cardiac tumors

Tumors of the heart muscle or surrounding tissues can result in cardiac dysfunction either by conduction irregularities or by mechanical interference secondary to pericardial effusion. Radiographs may reveal an enlarged and round heart shadow. Ultrasound may identify fluid accumulations or masses. When pericardial effusion is seen, aspiration of the fluid may reveal important diagnostic information. Although infrequent, tumors in the heart can be primary (hemangiosarcoma, chemodectoma) or metastatic (hemangiosarcoma, malignant lymphoma, carcinoma, or other widely metastatic tumors not typically seen in the heart).

Hemangiosarcoma

Figure 6.1 is a left lateral radiograph of a canine thorax showing an enlarged heart.

Figure 6.2 demonstrates a canine pericardial effusion showing acute hemorrhage FNA. The presence of platelets and the lack of macrophages containing heme pigment indicate that this is acute hemorrhage. Acute hemorrhage in the pericardium may be a result of vascular injury in the heart or pericardium, coagulopathy, or a cardiac vascular tumor, but collection trauma and resulting iatrogenic hemorrhage must also be considered.

Figure 6.3 is a canine pericardial effusion FNA showing chronic hemorrhage. The lack of platelets and the presence of macrophages containing heme pigment (arrows) indicate that this is chronic hemorrhage. This could be from a resolving prior transient hemorrhage or an ongoing persistent lesion such as hemangiosarcoma.

Figure 6.4 shows a biopsy of a canine myocardial hemangiosarcoma. A right atrial tumor was diagnosed by ultrasound in an 8-year-old intact male Labrador Retriever. Hemangiosarcoma was suspected, and euthanasia was elected. The specimen was a globoid heart with an enlarged, firm, mottled tan/red/black, thickened micronodular right atrium. On cut section a multinodular mass and blood clots filled the right atrium. Representative sections were processed for histopathology. In viable areas the mass was composed of moderately pleomorphic medium-sized polygonal and plump spindloid cells that formed solid aggregates and anastomosing capillary and sometimes cavernous blood-filled spaces. There was substantial replacement of the cardiac muscle wall of the right atrium. Hemosiderin-laden macrophages in the scant stroma indicated past hemorrhage. Mitoses were seen in the neoplastic endothelial cell population at a rate of 0–1/HPF, and some cells had double or multiple nuclei. Thus, the clinical diagnosis of hemangiosarcoma of the right atrium was confirmed. Right atrium is one of the most common sites for primary canine hemangiosarcoma, although these neoplasms are often multicentric by the time they are discovered. Infarction, hemorrhage, atrial rupture, and cardiac tamponade are common causes of death from this cardiac neoplasm.

Malignant plasma cell tumor

Figure 6.5 shows a cutaneous manifestation of a malignant plasma cell tumor in a dog. An aged neutered male Cocker Spaniel dog presented with multiple skin masses. Aspirate of a skin mass revealed a mixed population of typical plasma cells with an eosinophilic border, clumped chromatin, and scattered multinucleate cells. Cells with multiple nuclei exhibiting mild anisokaryosis are present in most plasma cell tumors and cannot be used to indicate prognosis.

Atlas for the Diagnosis of Tumors in the Dog and Cat, First Edition. Anita R. Kiehl and Maron Brown Calderwood Mays.
© 2016 John Wiley & Sons, Inc. Published 2016 by John Wiley & Sons, Inc.

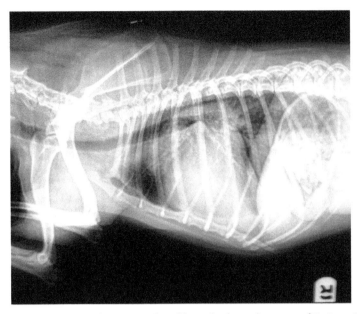

Figure 6.1 Left lateral radiograph of a canine thorax showing an enlarged heart. (Radiograph courtesy of Dr. Laura Hokett.)

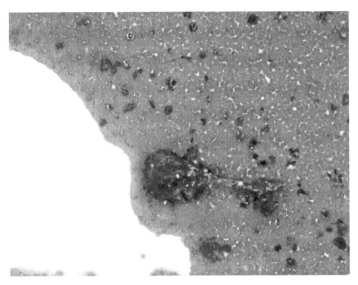

Figure 6.2 Canine pericardial effusion with acute hemorrhage FNA. 10x.

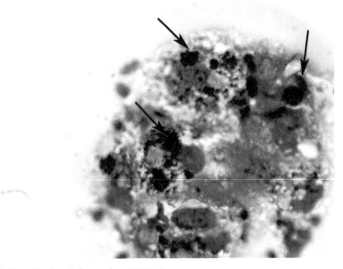

Figure 6.3 Canine pericardial effusion with chronic hemorrhage FNA. 40x.

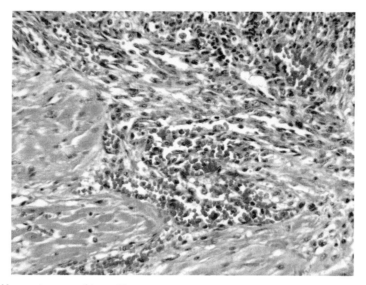

Figure 6.4 Canine myocardial hemangiosarcoma biopsy. 20x.

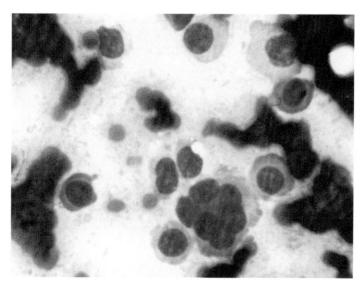

Figure 6.5 FNA of a cutaneous manifestation of malignant plasma cell tumor in a dog. 50x.

There can be cells with marked nuclear pleomorphism and giant lobulated nuclei in benign plasmacytoma. In this case the tumor was malignant, invaded multiple internal organs including the heart, and caused a fatal cardiac arrhythmia in the patient, as described in Figures 6.6 and 6.7, shown below.

Figure 6.6 shows canine pericardial effusion due to malignant plasma cell tumor metastatic to the heart FNA. This sample was collected postmortem at the same time as the sample shown in Figure 6.7. The amphophilic (both baso-philic and eosinophilic) cytoplasm of the cell at the lower left suggests plasma cell lineage. Multilobular nuclei are a hallmark of plasma cell tumor, but these nuclei exhibit marked anisokaryosis, clumped chromatin, and prominent nuclei within a deeply basophilic cytoplasm, which gives these cells a more aggressive appearance than the multinu-cleate cells from the skin mass in the same patient.

Figure 6.7 shows a postmortem biopsy of malignant plasma cell tumor metastatic to the heart in a dog. This adult neutered male Cocker Spaniel presented in ventricular fibrillation with a complaint of "not feeling well" and expired before lab work could be performed. Multiple cutaneous masses compatible with plasma cell tumor were seen on original presentation 1 week prior to the terminal event, but the owner declined workup. On necropsy there were white plaques and nodules throughout the heart and abdominal viscera, and the atypical cells infiltrating the myocardium are morphologically similar to the cells seen in multiple tissues in this patient. When a patient with disseminated neoplasia exhibits signs of cardiac disease, cardiac metastasis should be considered and appropriate diagnostic procedures performed, even if the tumor is not one typically associated with metastasis to the heart.

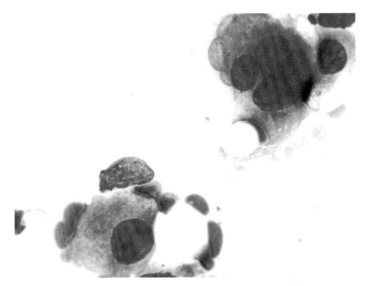

Figure 6.6 FNA of pericardial effusion in a dog due to malignant plasma cell tumor metastatic to the heart. 50x.

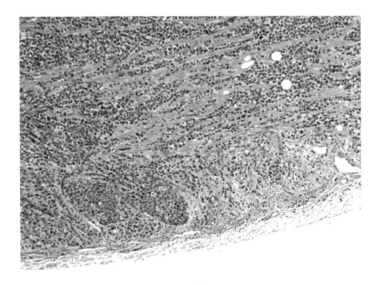

Figure 6.7 Biopsy of a postmortem sample of malignant plasma cell tumor metastatic to the heart in a dog. 10x.

Pulmonary mass lesions

Pulmonary disease can result in respiratory distress, which should lead to radiographic evaluation. When radiographs reveal pulmonary masses, look for thoracic cavity effusion. Cytologic evaluation of an effusion can lead to a rapid diagnosis when clearly malignant cells are identified. If there is no effusion, ultrasound-guided FNA of a mass may allow rapid diagnosis.

Pulmonary carcinoma

Figure 6.8 shows a lateral thoracic radiograph with scattered pulmonary nodules suggestive of neoplasia.

Figure 6.9 shows FNA of a canine pleural effusion as a result of carcinoma. Aspirate of a pleural effusion in an adult female mixed breed dog showed atypical epithelioid cells with marked anisokaryosis suggesting a diagnosis of carcinoma. Note that the nuclei of this cluster of atypical cells are much larger than adjacent neutrophils, and the associated macrophages and mesothelial cells do not exhibit this marked variation in nuclear size.

Figure 6.10 shows a canine pulmonary carcinoma FNA. Ultrasound-guided aspiration of a pulmonary mass in an adult female dog revealed epithelioid cells with marked anisokaryosis, prominent nucleoli, and variably basophilic cytoplasm. This triad of malignant characteristics is suggestive of carcinoma.

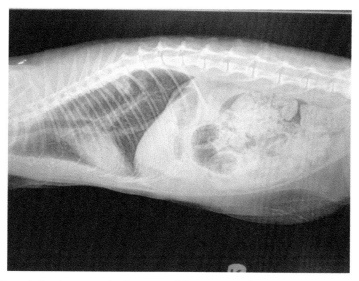

Figure 6.8 Lateral thoracic radiograph showing scattered pulmonary nodules suggestive of neoplasia. (Radiograph courtesy of Dr. Laura Hokett.)

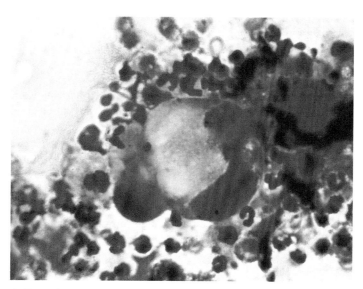

Figure 6.9 FNA of canine pleural effusion due to carcinoma. 50x.

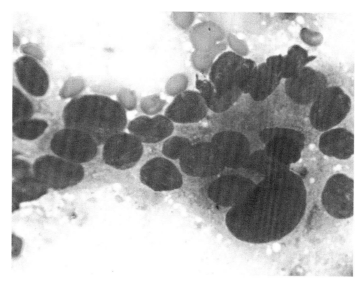

Figure 6.10 Canine pulmonary carcinoma FNA. 50x.

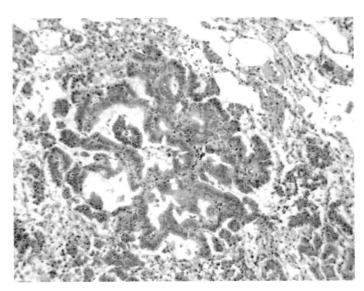

Figure 6.11 Canine pulmonary adenocarcinoma biopsy. 10x.

Figure 6.11 shows a biopsy of a canine pulmonary adenocarcinoma. A 14-year-old spayed female Borzoi had a lung mass on chest radiographs, which was a suspected lung tumor or possibly a pulmonary fungal infection. Three specimens were submitted in formalin and processed. The mass effacing much of the lung parenchyma in two specimens was a multilobular epithelial neoplasm comprised of branching tubules lined by crowded, enlarged, somewhat pleomorphic columnar cells that are often pseudostratified. The cells had surface blebs and microvilli. There was chronic lymphocytic and plasma cellular inflammation in portions of the stroma. Intralymphatic/intravascular embolization was not documented. Based on cytology and proliferative pattern, primary pulmonary adenocarcinoma was diagnosed. Metastatic adenocarcinoma is a histologic differential, but no other masses were discovered, and there was no history of an adenocarcinoma elsewhere (mammary, other.) Primary pulmonary adenocarcinomas can be multicentric in the lung by the time they are discovered, because they can spread elsewhere via lymphatics, blood vessels, and airways.

Pulmonary hemangiosarcoma
Figure 6.12 shows a canine pulmonary hemangiosarcoma FNA. Ultrasound-guided aspiration of a focal pulmonary lesion in an adult intact male Weimaraner revealed rare atypical spindloid to epithelioid cells with marked anisokaryosis in a background of blood. Most pulmonary aspirates yield scant to moderate blood due to the vascular nature of the lung. Neoplastic endothelial cells usually shed poorly on FNA so if even one cell with this degree of nuclear pleomorphism is seen on an aspirate neoplasia should be considered as a potential diagnosis. The definitive diagnosis is made by histologic evaluation.

Figure 6.13 shows a biopsy of a canine pulmonary hemangiosarcoma. A 10-year-old spayed female Bichon Frise was presented for "not feeling well." She had been anorexic at home and was trembling. Thoracic radiographs revealed lesions suggestive of metastatic disease, and euthanasia was elected. Necropsy revealed pulmonary metastases and a right-sided heart tumor. There were multiple nodules of varied size in the lung, and the lung tissue sank in fixative. The heart muscle also had nodules. There were coalescing multifocally hemorrhagic and necrotic nodules effacing the pulmonary parenchyma. The necrotic centers of these nodules often contained degenerate neutrophils. In viable areas the neoplastic nodules are composed of pleomorphic polygonal cells with marked variation in the size of the cells and their nuclei, one to three large nucleoli, and a moderate amount of eosinophilic cytoplasm. The mitotic rate was fairly high, and some cells have more than one nucleus. The neoplastic cells are arranged mostly in vague coalescing aggregates and sheets. There were hemorrhages within the nodules. The surrounding lung tissue exhibited severe proliferative interstitial pneumonitis. Emboli of neoplastic cells were found in capillaries and lymphatics. The neoplasm effacing the myocardium was identical to that disseminating throughout the lung, and there were tumor emboli in vessels throughout the myocardium. This neoplasm is a poorly differentiated hemangiosarcoma. These tumors can be primary in many tissues, and they metastasize readily via both blood vessels and lymphatics.

Pulmonary adenomatosis
Figure 6.14 shows a left lateral thoracic radiograph of a feline showing diffuse to nodular infiltrative disease typical of progressive histiocytic infiltrates.

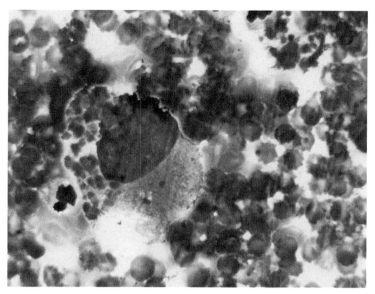

Figure 6.12 Canine pulmonary hemangiosarcoma FNA. 10x.

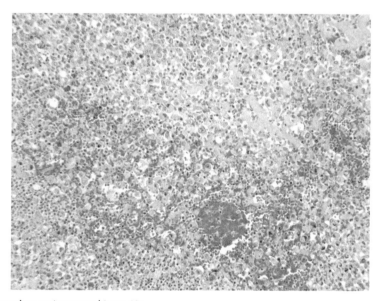

Figure 6.13 Canine pulmonary hemangiosarcoma biopsy. 10x.

Figure 6.15 shows feline pulmonary adenomatosis FNA. Aspiration of a lung mass in an adult neutered male cat with severe respiratory distress revealed many active macrophages in a background of scattered neutrophils and erythrocytes. The macrophages exhibit minimal anisokaryosis with small nucleoli typical of reactive cells. No infectious agents are seen. This type of mixed population can be seen with chronic inflammation secondary to infectious diseases and heart disease, or can be idiopathic.

Figure 6.16 shows a biopsy of a feline pulmonary adenomatosis. A 9-year-old neutered male Domestic Longhair cat had a 1-year history of severe respiratory disease that was diagnosed as pulmonary adenocarcinoma and type II pneumocyte hyperplasia at necropsy. A second opinion was requested, as this patient had no prior history of neoplasia in the lung or elsewhere, and there was no evidence of neoplasia or discrete tumor masses in the lung at the time of necropsy. This cat had a rare progressive incurable pulmonary disease that has had several names: pulmonary adenomatosis, chronic proliferative interstitial pneumonitis with multifocal adenomatosis, pulmonary carcinomatosis, feline pulmonary fibrosis (fibrosis is often not a feature), as well as other names. Note the proliferating enlarged cuboidal to columnar pneumocytes falling off the alveolar septa into the alveoli and airways. The disease is similar clinically,

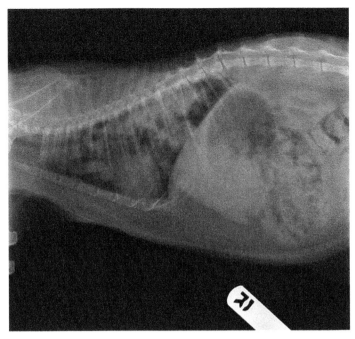

Figure 6.14 Left lateral thoracic radiograph of a feline showing diffuse to nodular infiltrative disease typical of progressive histiocytic infiltrates. (Radiograph courtesy of Dr. Barbara Larsen.)

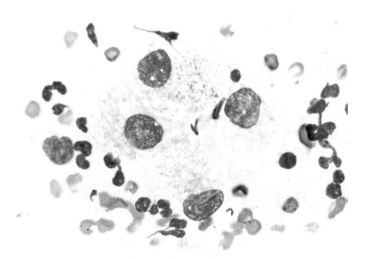

Figure 6.15 Feline pulmonary adenomatosis FNA. 40x.

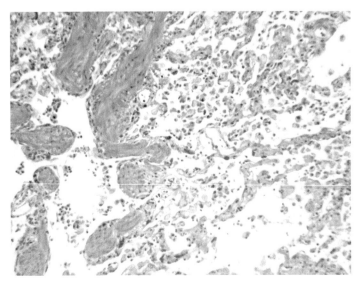

Figure 6.16 Feline pulmonary adenomatosis biopsy. 10x.

grossly, and histologically to jaagziekte/ovine pulmonary adenocarcinoma in sheep, which is caused by a retrovirus. In cats the lesions may be localized, multicentric, or fairly diffuse throughout all lung lobes. The etiology in felines is unknown. Potential causes of these progressive proliferative changes include viral infection and inhalation, ingestion, or percutaneous absorption of a pulmonary toxin.

Mediastinal tumors

Radiographic evaluation of an animal in respiratory distress may reveal a dense mass in the anterior chest in the area of the mediastinum. The structures most likely to cause a mass of this type are thymus and mediastinal lymph nodes. Masses in this area may cause pleural cavity effusion, and FNA of this effusion may be diagnostic. If there is no effusion, ultrasound-guided FNA of the mass is suggested as a useful diagnostic tool.

Figure 6.17 shows a feline left lateral thoracic radiograph showing a mediastinal mass.

Mediastinal malignant lymphoma
Figure 6.18 shows an FNA of a feline pleural effusion. Aspirate of fluid free in the thoracic cavity of a 2-year-old male cat with respiratory distress showed atypical lymphocytes compatible with lymphosarcoma. Note the reactive mesothelial cell (arrow) with a typical fringe border and the neutrophil. These lymphocytes are larger than the neutrophil, have fine to clumped chromatin with occasional nucleoli, and have moderate, light basophilic, vacuolated cytoplasm. A few

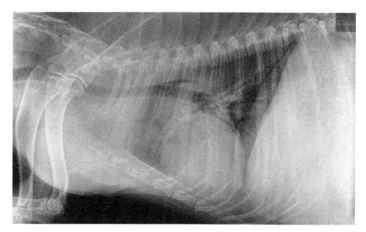

Figure 6.17 Feline left lateral thoracic radiograph showing a mediastinal mass. (Radiograph courtesy of Dr. Laura Hokett.)

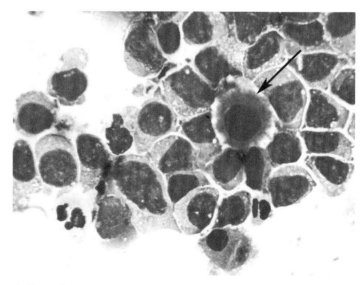

Figure 6.18 FNA of feline pleural effusion showing atypical lymphocytes compatible with lymphosarcoma. 50x.

small to medium lymphocytes are present. Ultrasonography could be helpful to look for a mediastinal mass that could be aspirated for confirmatory testing. Mediastinal lymphoma can cause enough fluid buildup to mask the inciting mediastinal neoplasm on radiographs, therefore, ultrasound should be considered when evaluating a patient with pleural effusion. This neoplasm is often associated with feline leukemia virus (FeLV) infection, and viral serology is recommended for optimization of treatment options and a more comprehensive prognosis.

Figure 6.19 shows a feline mediastinal malignant lymphoma FNA. Ultrasound-guided aspiration of a mediastinal mass found in a 2-year-old male neutered cat with respiratory distress revealed a dense population of round cells larger than the neutrophil, nucleoli are seen in cells with an intact cytoplasmic membrane, and there is scant to moderate basophilic cytoplasm. There is a mitotic figure in the lower left quadrant (arrow). Note that there are broken cells with what appear to be nucleoli. The expansion of chromatin in broken cells can mimic a nucleolus, and thus interpretation of broken cells should be avoided.

Figure 6.20 shows a feline mediastinal malignant lymphoma biopsy. A 4-year-old neutered male Domestic Shorthair cat was presented with severe respiratory distress and a possible mass in the chest. Euthanasia was elected. At necropsy there was excess fluid in the chest and a 3- x 2-inch thoracic mass suspected to be lymphoma. Fixed mass, heart, and lung sections were submitted. The photomicrograph is from the thoracic mass. It was diagnosed as malignant

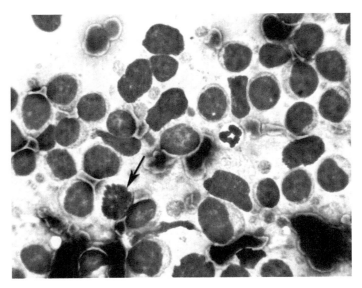

Figure 6.19 Feline mediastinal malignant lymphoma FNA. 10x.

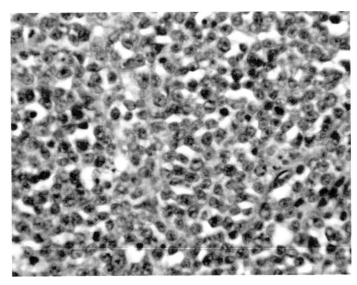

Figure 6.20 Feline mediastinal malignant lymphoma biopsy. 40x.

lymphoma, high grade, diffuse pattern, mixed medium and large cell types, with a low-intermediate mitotic rate. No lymph node or thymic architecture was recognized histologically. The mass is comprised of sheets of pleomorphic yet homogeneous polygonal and round cells that appear lymphoid. Nuclei vary from 1.0–2.0 X red blood cell size. The largest nuclei have a large nucleolus. Other cells have multiple smaller nucleoli. Mitoses were seen at a rate of 0–4/HPF, depending on the area. The clinical diagnosis of malignant lymphoma in the thoracic cavity was thus confirmed. The respiratory distress was caused by collapse of all but the caudal-most lung lobes due to this space-occupying lesion. Malignant lymphoma is a multicentric disease eventually, but it can start as a solitary mass in the thorax, either in the thymus or the anterior mediastinal lymph nodes.

Thymoma

Figure 6.21 shows a canine thymoma FNA. Aspirate of a canine thymoma can show mostly small to medium lymphocytes. Biopsy would be necessary to differentiate thymoma from a reactive lymph node or lymphocytic neoplasia.

Figure 6.22 shows a canine thymoma biopsy. A 7-1/2-year-old spayed female Maremma Sheepdog was presented with recent drastic weight loss and eating very little. Thoracic radiographs revealed a large mass in the anterior mediastinum pressing on the esophagus. A 2-pound mass with necrotic center was removed from the anterior mediastinum.

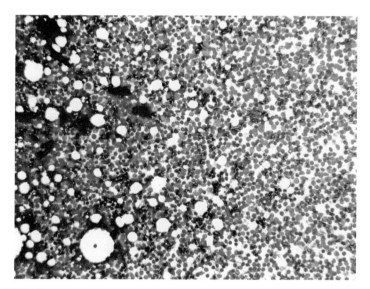

Figure 6.21 Canine thymoma FNA. 10x.

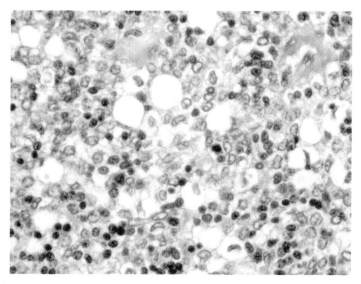

Figure 6.22 Canine thymoma biopsy. 10x.

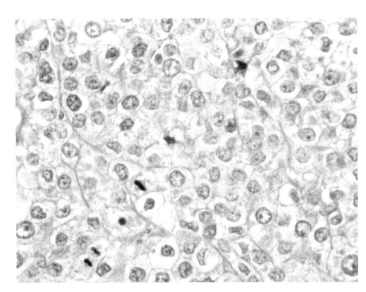

Figure 6.23 Canine malignant thymoma biopsy. 40x.

No metastases were seen in the lungs or intrathoracic lymph nodes. The mass was divided into irregular lobules by fibrous connective tissue septa. The epithelial cells are arranged in sheets and vague coalescing packets. The predominant cell type is a medium-sized, fairly uniform, polygonal epithelial cell with a medium-sized round nucleus, marginated chromatin, and small nucleoli. Cytoplasm is moderate in amount and eosinophilic or clear, foamy, or faintly granular. Mitotic figures were not seen after a moderate search. The epithelial cells occasionally lined small cysts. Hassall's corpuscles were not recognized, but dispersed among the epithelial components were aggregates of small lymphocytes. The touch preparation contained two cell types, small lymphocytes and uniform larger round cells similar to the epithelial cells seen on histology.

Figure 6.23 shows a canine recurrent thymoma biopsy. The mass recurred a year later. This time there was no lymphocytic component. The mass is comprised of sheets of medium-sized polygonal cells with moderate variation in nuclear size, multiple small or indistinct nucleoli, and a moderate amount of eosinophilic or vacuolated cytoplasm. Modest numbers of mitotic figures were seen. Ischemic necrosis and cystic degeneration were multifocal, but this was not a prominent finding. No metastases were recognized, but euthanasia was elected because of the development of malignant cytologic features and the high risk of another recurrence.

Additional reading

Thompson CA, Rebar AH. Body Cavity Effusions. In Canine and Feline Cytology; A Color Atlas and Interpretation Guide. 3rd ed. Raskin and Meyer. 2016. Elsevier. St. Louis. 191–219.

Cardiac tumors

Robinson WF, Robinson NA. Cardiovascular System. In Jubb, Kennedy, and Palmer's Pathology of Domestic Animals. Vol 3. 6th ed. M. Grant Maxie, Editor. Elsevier. St Louis. 2016. 1–101.
Kisseberth, WC. Neoplasia of the Heart. In Small Animal Clinical Oncology, 5th ed. Withrow and MacEwen. 2013. Elsevier. St. Louis. 700–706.

Hemangiosarcoma
Morrison WB. Hemangiosarcoma, Heart. In Blackwell's Five-Minute Veterinary Consult: Canine and Feline. 5th ed. Tilley LP and Smith FWK, Jr. 2011. John Wiley & Sons, Inc. West Sussex, UK. 543.

Pulmonary mass lesions

Burkhard MJ. Respiratory Tract. In Canine and Feline Cytology; A Color Atlas and Interpretation Guide. 3rd ed. Raskin and Meyer. 2016. Elsevier. St. Louis. 138–190.

Caswell JL, Williams KJ. Respiratory System. In Jubb, Kennedy, and Palmer's Pathology of Domestic Animals. Vol 2. 6th ed. M. Grant Maxie, Editor. Elsevier. St Louis. 2016. 465–591.

Grimes CN, Fry MM, LeBlanc CJ, Hecht S. The Lung and Intrathoracic Structures. In Cowell and Tyler's Diagnostic Cytology and Hematology of the Dog and Cat. 4th ed. Valenciano and Cowell. 2014. 291–311.

Rebhun RB, Culp WTN. Pulmonary Neoplasia. In Small Animal Clinical Oncology, 5th ed. Withrow and MacEwen. 2013. Elsevier. St. Louis. 453–462.

Pulmonary carcinoma

Selting KA. Adenocarcinoma, Lung. In Blackwell's Five-Minute Veterinary Consult: Canine and Feline. 5th ed. Tilley LP and Smith FWK, Jr. 2011. John Wiley & Sons, Inc. West Sussex, UK. 25.

Mediastinal tumors

Grimes CN, Fry MM, LeBlanc CJ, Hecht S. The Lung and Intrathoracic Structures. In Cowell and Tyler's Diagnostic Cytology and Hematology of the Dog and Cat. 4th ed. Valenciano and Cowell. 2014. 291–311.

Raskin RE. Hemolymphatic System. In Canine and Feline Cytology; A Color Atlas and Interpretation Guide. 3rd ed. Raskin and Meyer. 2016. Elsevier. St. Louis. 91–137.

Valli VEO, Kiupel M, Bienzle D. Hematopoietic System. In Jubb, Kennedy, and Palmer's Pathology of Domestic Animals. Vol 3. 6th ed. M. Grant Maxie, Editor. Elsevier. St Louis. 2016. 102–268.

Mediastinal malignant lymphoma

Morrison WB. Lymphoma-Dogs. In Blackwell's Five-Minute Veterinary Consult: Canine and Feline. 5th ed. Tilley LP and Smith FWK, Jr. 2011. John Wiley & Sons, Inc. West Sussex, UK. 778–779.

Selting KA. Lymphoma-Cats. In Blackwell's Five-Minute Veterinary Consult: Canine and Feline. 5th ed. Tilley LP and Smith FWK, Jr. 2011. John Wiley & Sons, Inc. West Sussex, UK. 776–77.

Vail D. Feline Lymphoma and Leukemia. In Small Animal Clinical Oncology, 5th ed. Withrow and MacEwen. 2013. Elsevier. St. Louis. 638–653.

Vail D, Pinkerton ME, Young KE. Canine Lymphoma and Lymphoid Leukemias. In Small Animal Clinical Oncology, 5th ed. Withrow and MacEwen. 2013. Elsevier. 608–638.

Thymoma

De Mello Souza CH. Thymoma. In Small Animal Clinical Oncology, 5th ed. Withrow and MacEwen. 2013. Elsevier. St. Louis. 688–691.

Selting KA. Thymoma. In Blackwell's Five-Minute Veterinary Consult: Canine and Feline. 5th ed. Tilley LP and Smith FWK, Jr. 2011. John Wiley & Sons, Inc. West Sussex, UK. 1231.

7 Selected Lesions of the Abdominal Viscera

Diseases that result in liver enlargement

The unexpected finding of abnormal serum levels of compounds related to hepatocellular homeostasis or function is often the first indication of liver disease. Elevations in serum alanine aminotransferase, alkaline phosphatase, bilirubin, gamma glutamate transferase, or bile acids can result in a search for underlying liver or metabolic disease in an apparently healthy patient. Changes in hepatic size and homogeneity noted on radiographs or ultrasound can be evaluated by FNA of the liver parenchyma. Vacuolar hepatopathy is a common result of hypercortisolism and can result in a markedly enlarged liver. Lesions such as regenerative nodules, hepatocellular neoplasia, lymphosarcoma, and bile duct neoplasia usually require biopsy for definitive diagnosis, but a presumptive diagnosis made by FNA can be useful to plan an appropriate diagnostic path. Vascular neoplasia requires biopsy for definitive diagnosis.

Vacuolar hepatopathy

Figure 7.1 is a canine abdominal radiograph showing an enlarged liver and spleen. This adult spayed female Maltese was being treated for immune mediated hemolytic anemia with high doses of corticosteroids, and the enlarged liver is typical of steroid hepatopathy.

Figure 7.2 shows a canine normal liver FNA. This cluster of typical hepatocytes exhibits small nuclei with mild anisokaryosis and lightly basophilic to amphophilic cytoplasm. The liver is a metabolically active organ so multiple small nucleoli and rare binucleate cells suggestive of a regenerative response can be seen in a healthy liver. These hepatocytes do not exhibit vacuolar change.

Figure 7.3 shows a canine vacuolar hepatopathy FNA. The foamy cytoplasm, seen in these clusters of hepatocytes in an adult female Maltese dog, can be described as hepatic vacuolar change. Variably sized vacuoles, affecting hepatocytes in a diffuse and widespread pattern, can be a result of systemic disease such as diabetes mellitus or hypercortisolism. Focal nodules of vacuolated hepatocytes can be seen with nodular regeneration, hepatocellular adenoma, and hepatocellular carcinoma. FNA cannot differentiate these etiologies. Biopsy is necessary to evaluate the hepatic architecture for a more accurate diagnosis of the disease process.

Bile duct hyperplasia

Figure 7.4 shows a canine hepatic bile duct hyperplasia FNA. An adult neutered male mixed breed dog presented with an elevated serum alkaline phosphatase level and radiographs revealed an enlarged liver. Hepatic aspiration revealed a background of blood with scattered neutrophils and small lymphocytes and clumps of typical hepatocytes (arrow) with smaller cuboidal ductular cells (arrowhead). There is minimal anisokaryosis, and the cells have scant cytoplasm typical of ductular epithelium. This cluster of duct-like cells would not be expected in normal tissue and, because there are monomorphic small nuclei, hyperplasia is the tentative cytologic diagnosis. This should be confirmed by biopsy as well-differentiated carcinoma can have this cytologic appearance.

Figure 7.5 shows a canine mild vacuolar hepatopathy with bile duct hyperplasia biopsy. A 4-year-old mixed breed dog died and was presented for necropsy. There was histologic evidence of severe chronic renal disease. Evaluation

Atlas for the Diagnosis of Tumors in the Dog and Cat, First Edition. Anita R. Kiehl and Maron Brown Calderwood Mays.
© 2016 John Wiley & Sons, Inc. Published 2016 by John Wiley & Sons, Inc.

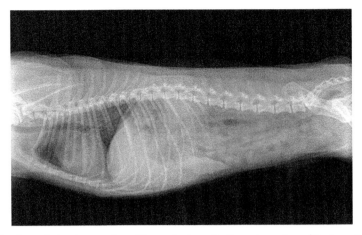

Figure 7.1 Canine abdominal radiograph showing an enlarged liver and spleen. (Radiograph courtesy of Dr. Laura Hokett.)

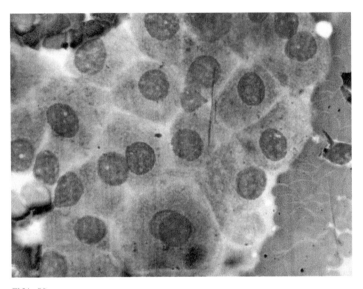

Figure 7.2 Canine normal liver FNA. 50x.

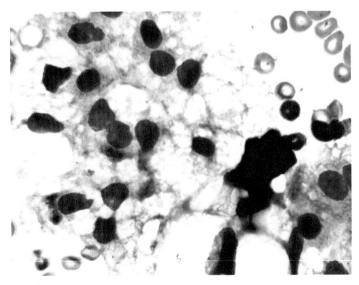

Figure 7.3 Canine vacuolar hepatopathy FNA. 50x.

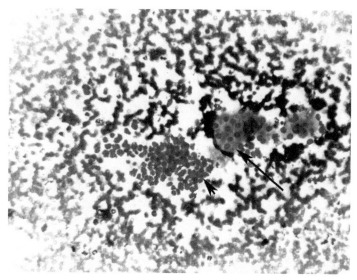

Figure 7.4 Canine hepatic bile duct hyperplasia FNA. 10x.

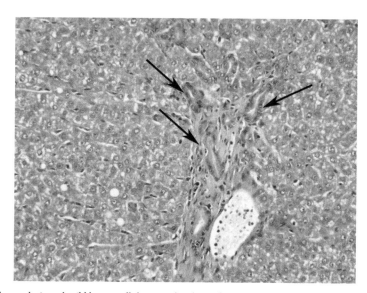

Figure 7.5 Canine bile duct hyperplasia and mild hepatocellular vacuolar change biopsy. 10x.

of the liver showed diffuse mild hepatocellular vacuolar change, a slightly nodular appearance to the architecture, and a portal proliferation of bile ducts lined by plump epithelium (arrows). Bile duct hyperplasia was diagnosed; the etiology was unknown.

Hepatocellular neoplasia

Figure 7.6 is a biopsy of a canine hepatoma. An 11-year-old spayed female Maltese presented with gastrointestinal signs. Abdominal ultrasound identified a 6-cm-diameter mass in the left lateral liver lobe. Exploratory celiotomy revealed that the mass was adhered to the stomach wall. The affected liver lobe was excised, as was a portion of the seromuscular layer of the stomach. Histologically the mass was deemed to be a hepatoma or very well-differentiated hepatocellular carcinoma with multifocal and coalescing ischemic necrosis. The mass was circumscribed but not encapsulated. It is composed of narrow trabeculae of well-differentiated hepatocytes with little variation in cell and nuclear size. It contains large irregular foci of ischemic necrosis, which are sometimes severely congested to hemorrhagic. Throughout the mass the hepatocytes sometimes contain lipid, and they exhibit mild vacuolar degeneration. MI = 0/10 HPF, and most cells are mononuclear although cells with double nuclei are present. There was some compression of the adjacent hepatic parenchyma, which exhibited moderate hemosiderosis and lipofuscinosis.

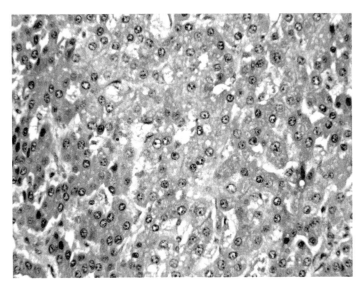

Figure 7.6 Canine hepatoma biopsy. 20x.

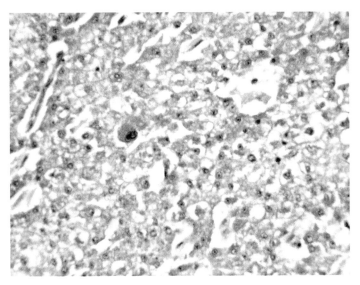

Figure 7.7 Canine hepatocellular carcinoma biopsy. 20x.

The large liver mass in this case had outgrown its blood supply, but the cells comprising it are still well differentiated with a low mitotic rate, and the mass was circumscribed, although not encapsulated. Thus, it is mostly likely a large hepatoma. However, it is difficult to differentiate hepatomas from well-differentiated hepatocellular carcinomas histologically. Complete resection could be curative, but careful follow-up was advised.

Figure 7.7 is a biopsy of a canine hepatocellular carinoma. An 11-year-old neutered male Labrador Retriever mix was presented for a few weeks of not feeling well. A large anterior abdominal mass was palpated. Exploratory laparotomy revealed a friable 25-cm irregular round mass involving the left medial liver lobe. It was surgically excised, and selected sections were fixed in formalin and submitted for histopathology. It was a fairly well-differentiated hepatocellular carcinoma with multifocal ischemic and hemorrhagic necrosis, cystic degeneration, and hemorrhage. In viable areas the mass is comprised of somewhat pleomorphic medium-sized polygonal hepatocytes that often suffer vacuolar degeneration with some lipidosis. There is moderate variation in cell and nuclear size. Most cells are mononuclear. Scattered cells with more than one nucleus are seen. Occasional mitotic figures were noted in this cell population. The cells are arranged in vague coalescing aggregates, sheets, and irregular cords, lacking portal triads. Some compressed hepatic parenchyma along the periphery was fibrotic, and the entrapped hepatocytes there suffered severe vacuolar degeneration. Timely complete resection can be curative. However, these tumors are capable of recurrence after resection, they can eventually metastasize via blood vessels and lymphatics, and they occasionally seed the abdomen.

Bile duct carcinoma

Figure 7.8 shows FNA of a feline bile duct carcinoma. A 15-year-old female Domestic Shorthair cat was presented for anorexia and weight loss. Radiographs revealed an enlarged liver, and an ultrasound-guided aspiration was performed. The aspirate revealed pleomorphic epithelial cells exhibiting marked anisokaryosis, prominent nucleoli and basophilic, and occasionally finely vacuolated cytoplasm. This suggests a diagnosis of carcinoma. Biopsy is necessary to determine the tissue of origin.

Figure 7.9 shows a canine cholangiocarcinoma biopsy. A 15-year-old neutered male Yorkshire Terrier was presented for acute vomiting, diarrhea, rapid weight loss, and changes in behavior. Necropsy samples of liver were submitted, as the liver had nodules. There were multiple masses and nodules disrupting the hepatic parenchyma. They are composed of moderately pleomorphic medium to large polygonal epithelial cells with considerable variation in cell and nuclear size, a large nucleus with one or two prominent nucleoli, and a moderate amount of eosinophilic cytoplasm. Mitoses were easily found in this cell population. The cells are arranged in sheets, closely packed cords, and they sometimes form tubules of varied diameter. Ischemic necrosis and cystic degeneration were multifocal. Throughout the compromised hepatic parenchyma there were numerous large aggregates of hemosiderin-laden macrophages, as well. The nodules varied considerably in size. Since no neoplasms were recognized elsewhere, this neoplasm was believed to be of bile duct origin. Biliary carcinomas are often multicentric by the time they are discovered, and they can metastasize both via blood vessels and lymphatics.

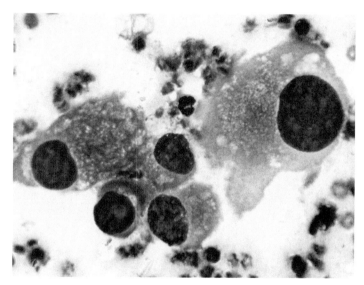

Figure 7.8 Feline bile duct carcinoma FNA. 50x.

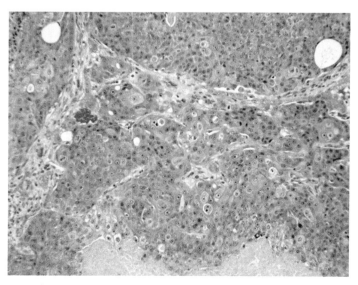

Figure 7.9 Canine cholangiocarcinoma biopsy. 10x.

Hepatic hemangiosarcoma

Figure 7.10 shows a canine hepatic hemangiosarcom FNA. An adult male Weimaraner dog presented for a pendulous abdomen. Aspiration revealed free blood. Euthanasia was performed and an impression was made of a liver mass. In a background of blood, large platelet clumps, and increased neutrophils, there are clusters of typical hepatocytes (arrowhead) and scattered large epithelioid cells with marked anisokaryosis, prominent nucleoli, and basophilic wispy cytoplasm (arrows). The blood and platelet clumps indicate acute hemorrhage, which is typical of, but not diagnostic for, vascular tumors. The inflammation suggests tissue necrosis. The pleomorphic cells are likely neoplastic cells. Histopathology revealed hemangiosarcoma. FNA of the liver antemortem would likely have yielded only blood, but finding even a few pleomorphic cells with this appearance would strongly suggest sarcomatous neoplasia.

Figure 7.11 shows a canine hepatic hemangiosarcoma biopsy. A spayed female mixed breed canine of unknown age was presented with hemoabdomen and bleeding liver nodules. A liver nodule was submitted. The poorly circumscribed mass is comprised of pleomorphic polygonal and plump spindloid vascular endothelial cells that form anastomosing blood-filled spaces. Clotted blood was adherent to the liver capsule in this area. The remainder of the liver exhibited

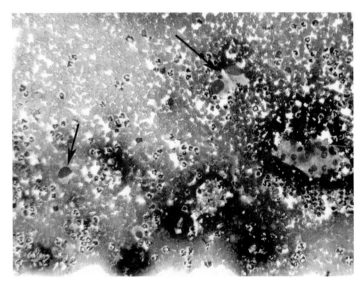

Figure 7.10 Canine hepatic hemangiosarcoma FNA. 10x.

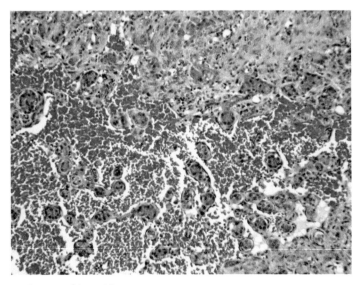

Figure 7.11 Canine hepatic hemangiosarcoma biopsy. 10x.

moderate vacuolar degeneration of hepatocytes. Hemangiosarcomas are frequently multicentric within the abdomen by the time they are discovered. They can be primary at almost any site in the body, and within the abdomen they often seed the abdomen, whether of splenic, hepatic, or other tissue origin. They also metastasize readily via both blood vessels and lymphatics.

Gastrointestinal lesions

A mass in the intestine can often easily be evaluated by FNA. A search for an abdominal effusion that could be evaluated cytologically is a prudent first step as penetration of the intestine, or an intestinal neoplasm, may not be necessary if FNA of the effusion is diagnostic. Peritoneal fluid FNA is also a great help to look for free infectious agents in the peritoneum. Lymphoplasmacellular and eosinophilic inflammatory infiltrates in the intestinal mucosa can mimic a mass. FNA can give a preliminary diagnosis, but biopsy is usually recommended for definitive diagnosis. Those disease processes, however, are typically more amenable to medical therapy than surgical excision, and FNA may offer a diagnostic approach less intrusive than surgery as a first step.

Eosinophilic inflammatory bowel disease

Figure 7.12 shows canine eosinophilic inflammatory bowel disease FNA. Aspiration of an intestinal mass that yields 25% or greater eosinophils is suggestive of eosinophilic inflammatory bowel disease. This disease may be a response to dietary or parasitic antigens, and medical therapy is warranted prior to biopsy. Eosinophilia can be a paraneoplastic response to lymphoma or carcinoma, so persistence of clinical signs despite therapy would be an indication for biopsy.

Figure 7.13 shows a biopsy of canine eosinophilic inflammatory bowel disease. This 7-year-old neutered male mix breed dog presented with uncontrollable diarrhea. Eosinophilic inflammatory bowel disease consists of recognizable infiltrates of eosinophils in the lamina propria, often with superficial ulceration and scattered infiltrates of neutrophils, small lymphocytes, and plasma cells. Perivascular eosinophilic infiltrates can sometimes be seen in the submucosa. Granulomatous lesions extending into the submucosa and muscular layers (layers not seen on this biopsy) are suspicious for invasive infectious organisms such as *Pythium sp.* and appropriate additional tests, such as Gomori Methenamine Silver (GMS) fungal stain of the biopsy or serology for fungal antigens, should be considered.

Lymphoplasmacellular inflammatory bowel disease

Figure 7.14 shows an FNA of feline lymphoplasmacellular inflammatory bowel disease. Aspirate of a thickened bowel wall in an adult neutered male Siamese cat revealed a population composed of small to medium lymphocytes, plasma cells and scattered neutrophils, macrophages, and rare large lymphocytes. This is compatible with an inflammatory process. Lymphocytic neoplasia can arise from sites of chronic lymphoid hyperplasia, so additional testing such as flow cytometry to look for a monomorphic cell type, antigen receptor site rearrangement polymerase chain reaction (PCR) to look for clonality, or biopsy may be necessary for a more definitive diagnosis. If a diffuse inflammatory process is suspected based on radiographs and ultrasound-guided FNA, complete excision of the lesion might not be indicated or even possible, and medical therapy could be the appropriate therapeutic plan.

Figure 7.15 shows a feline lymphoplasmacellular inflammatory bowel disease biopsy. A young adult spayed female Domestic Shorthair cat presented with chronic diarrhea unresponsive to treatment. Lymphoplasmacellular inflammatory bowel disease can be diagnosed by finding villi expanded by variably dense mixed inflammatory infiltrates of small lymphocytes and plasma cells that are confined to the lamina propria, often with preservation of the overlying epithelial layer and dilation of villus lacteals. PARR (PCR for antigen receptor site rearrangement) could be helpful to exclude an emerging population of clonal lymphocytes.

Gastrointestinal malignant lymphoma

Figure 7.16 shows FNA of feline intestinal high-grade lymphosarcoma. An aged neutered male Domestic Shorthair cat was presented for anorexia and weight loss. Palpation revealed an intestinal mass. An aspirate revealed sheets of lymphoblasts, and a preliminary diagnosis of lymphosarcoma was made. There were frequent mitotic figures (upper right and lower left) that suggest a high-grade tumor. Lymphoid follicles are present in some areas of the intestine and may be quite large when associated with chronic inflammatory lesions so finding a few lymphoblasts is not diagnostic of malignant lymphoma and biopsy is recommended for definitive diagnosis.

Figure 7.17 shows a biopsy of a feline epitheliotropic lymphoma, gastric mucosa. An 11-year-old spayed female Calico cat had been vomiting on and off for 6 weeks. The gastric mucosa, duodenal mucosa, and a gastric lymph node

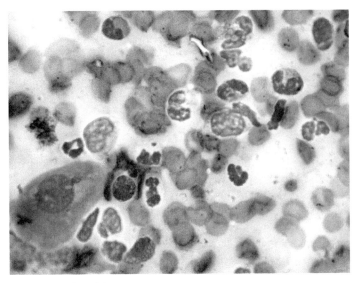

Figure 7.12 Canine eosinophilic inflammatory bowel disease FNA. 50x.

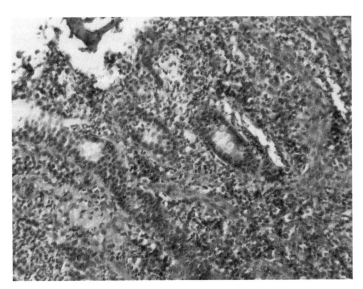

Figure 7.13 Canine eosinophilic inflammatory bowel disease biopsy. 10x.

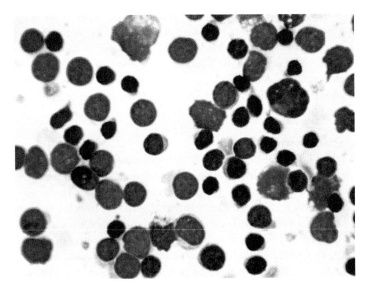

Figure 7.14 Feline lymphoplasmacellular inflammatory bowel disease FNA. 10x.

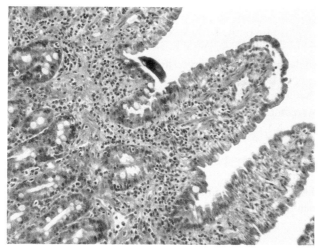

Figure 7.15 Feline lymphoplasmacellular inflammatory bowel disease biopsy. 10x.

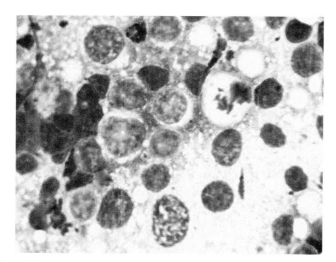

Figure 7.16 Feline intestinal high-grade lymphosarcoma FNA. 50x.

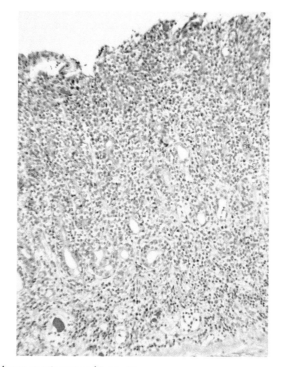

Figure 7.17 Feline epitheliotropic lymphoma, gastric mucosa biopsy. 40x.

were biopsied. The mucosal architecture of the body and fundus of the stomach are effaced by a diffuse infiltrate of enlarged lymphoid cells with enlarged nuclei, a central nucleolus, and scant cytoplasm. These cells are mononuclear. They infiltrate the gastric glandular mucosa extensively. The cells have nuclei up to 1.5 x red blood cell size, and mitotic figures were found in this cell population. The same cells infiltrated the gastric lymph node and the glands comprising the mucosa of the proximal duodenum. Because the enlarged lymphoid cells are epitheliotrophic, T-cell origin was suspected, but special stains were not done. Malignant lymphoma can be localized at first, but this is a multicentric disease eventually, involving multiple lymph nodes, spleen, liver, bone marrow, and peripheral blood.

Gastrointestinal adenocarcinoma

Figure 7.18 shows a feline intestinal adenocarcinoma with abdominal effusion FNA. A thin adult female Domestic Shorthair cat presented with a fluid-filled abdominal cavity that was found to have low cell counts and moderate levels of protein upon aspiration. Sedimentation of this peritoneal effusion, which was secondary to an intestinal adenocarcinoma, yielded many clusters of epithelioid cells with moderate to rare marked anisokaryosis, prominent nucleoli and basophilic cytoplasm with focal clearing suggestive of mucus production or fluid absorption by these free-floating cells. Finding of this type of cell cluster in the abdominal area allows a preliminary diagnosis of adenocarcinoma and advises that metastasis may have occurred, providing a useful data point for prognosis.

Figure 7.19 shows a biopsy of a canine small intestinal adenocarcinoma. A 3-year-old neutered male Standard Poodle had a history of vomiting and poor appetite for a few months. A mass was found in the small intestine. There was no intact mucosal surface on the intestinal section. What may have been mucosa in one area was fibrovascular tissue with infiltrating coalescing islands of pleomorphic medium to large polygonal epithelial cells with marked variation in cell and nuclear size, at least one large nucleolus, and a modest amount of pale cytoplasm. These cells form solid aggregates, closely packed trabeculae, and sometimes acinar and tubular structures lined by one to multiple layers of cells. Deeper in the wall there are infiltrative islands of these cells as well as dilated lymphatics containing tumor emboli. At least one vessel containing a tumor embolus also contains red blood cells. There was multifocal perivascular and nodular lymphoid follicular hyperplasia in the mesenteric attachment. Definitive intralymphatic embolization was not seen in the mesenteric attachment at the level examined. This intestinal mass is an invasive adenocarcinoma emanating from the mucosal lining of the small intestine. These tumors are locally aggressive, and many of them metastasize early to draining lymph nodes and then to more distant sites. The neoplasm had already invaded lymphatics and a vein locally. The patient seems young for this neoplasm.

Gastrointestinal spindle cell tumor

Figure 7.20 shows an FNA of an intestinal mass in an 11-year-old neutered male Labrador Retriever. The FNA revealed spindle cells in abnormally large clusters. There is moderate anisokaryosis and abundant wispy cytoplasm. A tumor of mesenchymal origin was suspected and biopsy recommended. Immunohistochemistry can then be performed on the biopsy section to identify the cell type, provide information for the best treatment protocol, and give a more accurate prognosis.

Figure 7.21 shows a biopsy of a canine gastrointestinal stromal tumor. A 5- to 6-cm-diameter round firm mass was found in the cecum on abdominal ultrasound. A typhlectomy was performed. Adenocarcinoma, leiomyosarcoma, and other diagnoses were ruled out. The liver was within normal limits. The cecal mass is comprised of short intersecting fascicles of pleomorphic polygonal and plump spindloid stromal cells. Nuclei vary in size. The cytoplasm is faintly granular and eosinophilic and streaming, with indistinct cell borders. Most cells are mononuclear. Scattered cells appear to have more than one nucleus, usually in a group. MI = 5/10 HPF. The neoplasm had infiltrated the adipose tissue of the mesenteric attachment. However, intralymphatic/intravascular embolization was not seen in the peripheral tissue available for examination. This is a gastrointestinal stromal tumor (GIST). Behavior is similar to that of a leiomyosarcoma, a pure smooth muscle tumor. These tumors can recur locally even if completely resected, and long distance metastasis to lymph nodes, liver, and spleen sometimes occurs, so consultation with an oncologist would be helpful for prognosis and the most current treatment protocol. There was no evidence of metastasis in the liver biopsy submitted.

Kidney and bladder masses

Kidney enlargement may be nodular or diffuse. In the cat, nodular to diffuse enlargement may be due to inflammation secondary to chronic Coronavirus infection (referred to as the granulomatous or "dry" form of feline infectious peritonitis or FIP). Diffuse enlargement in the cat or dog could be due to a neoplastic infiltrate of lymphocytes or a neoplastic proliferation of renal tubular epithelium.

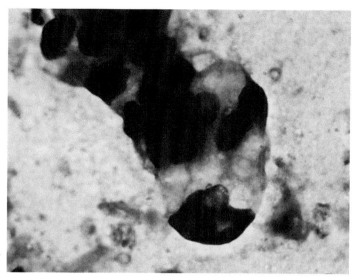

Figure 7.18 FNA of feline intestinal adenocarcinoma with abdominal effusion. 50x.

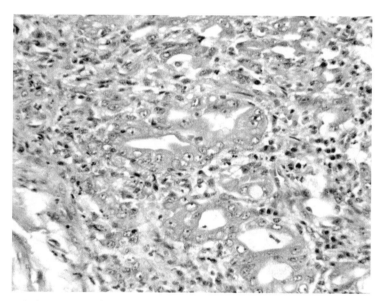

Figure 7.19 Canine small intestinal adenocarcinoma biopsy. 20x.

Pyogranulomatous inflammatory disease suggestive of feline infectious peritonitis

Figure 7.22 shows an FNA of feline kidney granuloma typical of FIP. An 11-month-old male Persian cat presented with fever, enlarged irregular kidneys, and early renal failure. Ultrasound-guided FNA of an enlarged and nodular kidney yielded clusters of active macrophages and neutrophils, with occasional small lymphocytes and plasma cells, a finding compatible with granuloma formation and suggestive of FIP. No infectious agents were seen on this aspirate. The clinical course of the disease was progressive and unresponsive to therapy, and the patient was humanely euthanized.

Figure 7.23 shows a biopsy of a feline kidney granuloma typical of FIP. Postmortem on the previously described 11-month-old male cat presented for fever and enlarged kidneys, revealed multifocal effacement of the normal renal tissue by nodules composed of perivascular active macrophages and neutrophils, around vessels with vasculitis and necrosis. There are scattered foci of small lymphocytes and plasma cells at the periphery of the nodules. The combination of ischemic necrosis secondary to vascular injury with the mass effect of the granulomas can result in renal dysfunction.

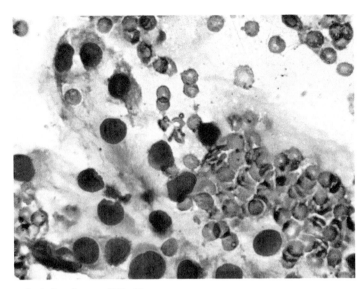

Figure 7.20 Canine gastrointestinal spindle cell tumor FNA. 50x.

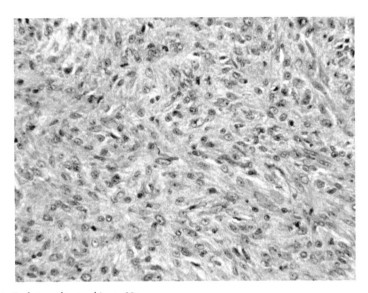

Figure 7.21 Canine gastrointestinal stromal tumor biopsy. 20x.

Renal carcinoma

Figure 7.24 shows FNA of a canine renal carcinoma. FNA of a large kidney mass in a 10-year-old neutered mixed breed dog revealed chains of monomorphic epithelial cells compatible with renal tubular epithelium. Aspiration of this number of cells is not a feature of a normal kidney, and a neoplastic proliferation of tubular epithelium was the preliminary diagnosis. Biopsy was recommended for definitive diagnosis.

Figure 7.25 shows a biopsy of a canine renal carcinoma. The left kidney of a 14-year-old neutered male mixed Cocker Spaniel was extremely enlarged with a necrotic center on gross evaluation. It exhibited ischemic and hemorrhagic necrosis and cystic degeneration within the renal cortex histologically. The mass is composed of moderately pleomorphic polygonal and cuboidal epithelial cells with moderate variation in nuclear size and a moderate amount of faintly granular eosinophilic cytoplasm. These cells line numerous tubules that are at times somewhat dilated. Pressure from the mass had incited a wide band of fibrous connective tissue in the adjacent renal parenchyma, accompanied by chronic inflammation, and there is extensive ischemic necrosis with hemorrhage and cystic degeneration in the center of the mass. The neoplastic cells are mostly mononuclear. Scattered cells have double nuclei. Nuclear size varies, but potential mitoses were infrequent throughout. Definitive intralymphatic and intravascular embolization was not

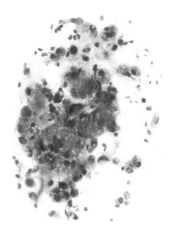

Figure 7.22 Feline kidney granuloma FNA. 10x.

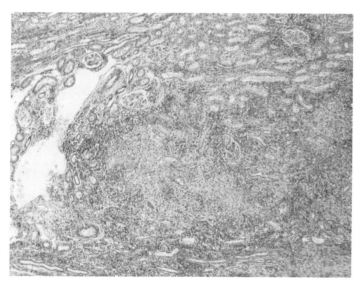

Figure 7.23 Feline kidney granuloma biopsy. 10x.

recognized in the areas chosen for histologic examination. This is a fairly well-differentiated epithelial neoplasm of renal tubular origin. It is sometimes difficult to differentiate benign from malignant varieties histologically, but these tumors are malignant in behavior much of the time in canines, and they are occasionally bilateral. Malignant varieties metastasize rather readily to draining lymph nodes and more distant organs, and they sometimes seed the abdomen. Further information was not available in this case.

Renal malignant lymphoma

Figure 7.26 shows an FNA of a feline renal lymphoma. A 12-year-old spayed female Domestic Shorthair cat presented with an enlarged kidney. Aspirate of this kidney yielded a dense population of medium to large lymphocytes with occasional lymphoblasts. Note dense clump of cells suggestive of glomerular tuft. There is not a significant resident population of lymphocytes in the kidney, so the preliminary diagnosis is malignant lymphoma (lymphosarcoma).

Figure 7.27 shows a biopsy of a feline renal lymphoma. A 13-year-old spayed female Domestic Shorthair cat died suddenly, and a necropsy was performed. Multifocal hemorrhagic lesions involved the kidneys, heart, mesentery, and mesenteric lymph nodes. Moderately pleomorphic medium-sized neoplastic cells with lymphoid features infiltrated

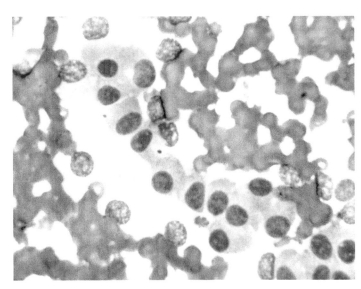

Figure 7.24 Canine renal carcinoma FNA. 50x.

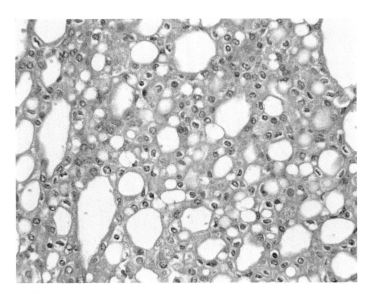

Figure 7.25 Canine renal carcinoma biopsy. 20x.

the renal cortex. The mitotic rate was considered to be intermediate grade. The renal lymphoma was interstitial, multinodular, and multifocal. The cells at multiple affected sites were consistent with fairly well-differentiated malignant lymphoma, which is usually a slowly progressive disease in felines that causes gradual weight loss and diarrhea. The cells at additional, probably newer, sites were more immature and less differentiated, as seen here.

Urinary bladder cystitis with reactive epithelial hyperplasia

Figure 7.28 shows FNA of canine bladder cystitis with reactive epithelium. Urine, collected by catheterization from a 10-year-old neutered male Bulldog, yielded a dense population of neutrophils, rare free and intracellular coccoid bacteria, and a population of epithelial cells, mostly individual or in small clumps, with plump nuclei, small nucleoli, and basophilic cytoplasm. These cells are metabolically active, as shown by the nucleoli and cytoplasmic basophilia, but this is a normal response to chronic bacterial infection and inflammation, as the nuclei in cells with an intact cytoplasmic membrane are only slightly larger than the neutrophils, and there is only mild anisokaryosis. Cytologic evaluation of cystitis due to uroliths, diverticulae, or polyps may have a similar epithelial appearance but may not exhibit this degree of inflammation or bacterial overgrowth.

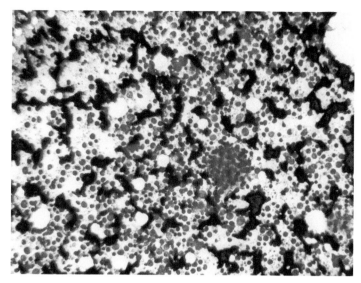

Figure 7.26 Feline renal lymphoma FNA. 10x.

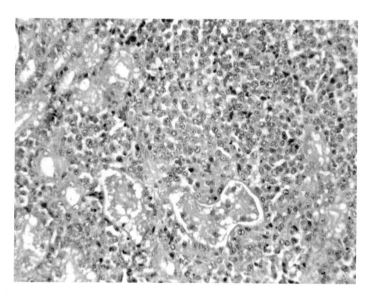

Figure 7.27 Feline renal lymphoma biopsy. 20x.

Figure 7.29 shows a biopsy of canine urinary bladder cystitis. A 6-year-old female French Bulldog presented for urinary incontinence, and radiographs revealed bladder stones. Biopsy samples were collected during cystotomy. Biopsy revealed ulceration of the mucosal epithelium with a population of metabolically active cells attempting to re-epithelialize the exposed and necrotic subepithelium. These active epithelial cells exhibit nuclei with clumped chromatin, prominent nucleoli, and abundant basophilic cytoplasm. There are neutrophils in the submucosa and infiltrating the variably necrotic epithelial layer.

Urinary bladder polyp

Figure 7.30 shows a biopsy of a canine urinary bladder polyp. A 15-year-old spayed female mixed breed dog presented with urinary incontinence, and radiographs revealed bladder stones. During cystotomy a pedunculated mass was noted and excised for biopsy. The epithelial layer of this proliferative polyp has a benign appearance with a thick wall of monomorphic epithelium, small nuclei, and a well-defined interface with no evidence of stromal invasion. Polyp formation can be a result of chronic trauma such as bladder stones or may be a developmental defect.

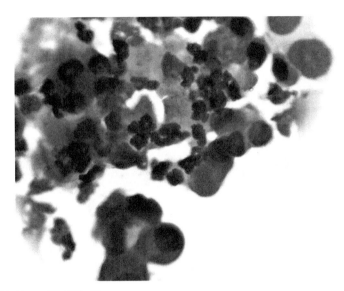

Figure 7.28 Canine urinary bladder cystitis FNA. 50x.

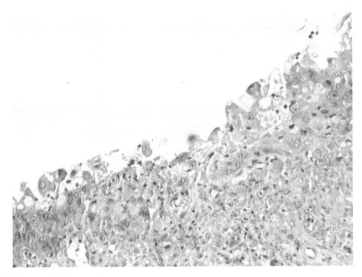

Figure 7.29 Canine urinary bladder cystitis biopsy. 10x.

Transitional cell carcinoma

Figure 7.31 shows canine bladder transitional cell carcinoma FNA. A 10-year-old male Bulldog presented with dysuria, and urine was collected by catherization. Cytologic exam reveals clusters of large epithelial cells with nuclei two to three times larger than a neutrophil, prominent nucleoli, and basophilic cytoplasm. The marked anisokaryosis is a hallmark of transitional cell carcinoma. If there is scant inflammation and no bacteria it decreases the possibility that the epithelial changes are due to reactive hyperplasia.

Figure 7.32 shows a feline bladder carcinoma biopsy. A 7-year-old neutered male Savannah cat had a chronic history of urinary tract infections. A radiograph revealed a solitary urolith. During surgery the bladder was noted to be thickened and firm, so two mucosal biopsies were submitted. An infiltrative carcinoma was diagnosed in one specimen. The other specimen consisted mostly of submucosa and smooth muscle, and it was not involved. The affected specimen is composed of dense fibrovascular tissue containing islands and anastomosing thick trabeculae of polygonal epithelial cells that are sometimes flattened or streaming. Definitive intercellular bridges are not recognized, and keratinization is not a feature. In one area presumed to be on the luminal surface, the luminal epithelium is multilayered and appears disorganized. Margins and depth of invasion could not be assessed. Urinary bladder epithelial neoplasms can recur even if completely resected and they metastasize via lymphatics.

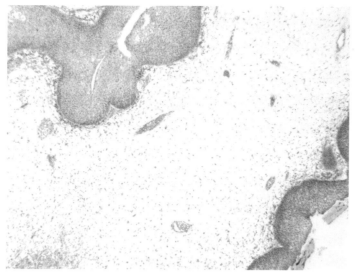

Figure 7.30 Canine urinary bladder polyp biopsy. 2.5x.

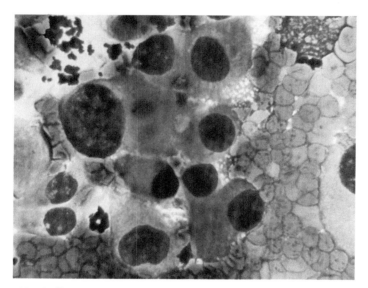

Figure 7.31 Canine bladder transitional cell carcinoma FNA. 50x.

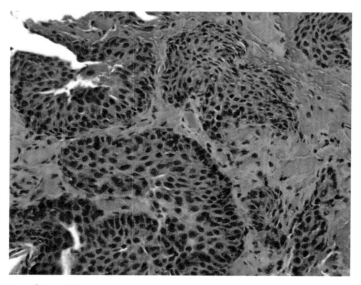

Figure 7.32 Feline bladder carcinoma biopsy. 20x.

Splenomegaly and splenic masses

Splenomegaly can be a result of proliferating normal splenic elements or can be due to a diffuse infiltrate of cells not normally present in high numbers in the spleen. Torsion or thrombosis of a major vein can result in splenomegaly due to congestion. Metastatic tumors can infiltrate the spleen in a nodular or diffuse pattern. Reactive populations can form small nodules and can then undergo malignant transformation to diffuse tumors.

Figure 7.33 shows a radiograph of a dog with splenomegaly. The spleen is homogeneous and suggests a diffuse infiltrate.

Extramedullary hematopoiesis

Figure 7.34 shows FNA of splenic extramedullary hematopoiesis. A 13-year-old spayed female Cocker Spaniel presented with hemolytic anemia. Radiographs revealed diffuse splenomegaly. Ultrasound-guided FNA revealed a proliferation of the normal population of developing hematopoietic elements including megakaryocytes (arrowhead), granulocytes (long arrow), and erythrocytes (medium arrow), which can result in diffuse splenomegaly. This may be a normal response to anemia or hypoxia.

Lymphoid nodular hyperplasia

Figure 7.35 shows a splenic nodule. This nodule was an incidental finding in a necropsy of a dog treated unsuccessfully for immune mediated hemolytic anemia. Fibrohistiocytic nodules and reactive lymphoid hyperplasia can produce nodules on the surface of the spleen that appear alarming on gross examination but are benign in behavior.

Figure 7.36 shows a splenic fibrohistiocytic nodule biopsy. A large splenic mass that appeared to have already ruptured at surgery was found in a 10-1/2-year-old neutered male Chihuahua, along with old free blood in abdomen. The mass was 4-1/2 cm in greatest dimension and was submitted in two pieces. Focal thrombosis was noted histologically, along with multifocal lymphoid nodular follicular hyperplasia, multifocal mild hemosiderosis, and abundant interstitial extramedullary hematopoiesis. It is partly cellular and partly more fibrous. A neoplastic cell population was not identified in the large representative sections chosen for histologic examination. The adjacent spleen exhibited acute passive congestion and abundant extramedullary hematopoiesis. This is a benign lesion that may be solitary or multicentric in the spleen. Thrombosis, hemorrhagic necrosis, and hemorrhage are common complications. Timely splenectomy is the treatment of choice. Malignant transformation to fibrosarcoma with metastasis to the liver has been reported, but is exceedingly rare.

Figure 7.37 shows canine splenic reactive lymphoid hyperplasia. Impression smears of the splenic nodule shown in Figure 7.35 revealed a mixed population of small to medium lymphocytes and scattered plasma cells with a few blasts. The interpretation of this population was reactive lymphoid hyperplasia.

Figure 7.38 shows a canine splenic lymphoid nodular hyperplasia biopsy. Histology was performed on the splenic nodule shown in Figure 7.36, revealing a large lymphoid follicle composed of a germinal center of lymphoblasts ringed by smaller lymphocytes and plasma cells. Immunohistochemistry could be used to identify B and T lymphocytes (see Chapter 8), and antigen receptor site rearrangement PCR could be used to look for clonality, which, if present, would suggest an emerging neoplastic process. Lymphoid neoplasia can develop from sites of reactive lymphoid populations.

Malignant lymphoma

Figure 7.39 shows a splenic lymphosarcoma FNA. Ultrasound-guided aspiration of an enlarged spleen in a 10-year-old female Maltese dog yielded a dense monomorphic population of large lymphocytes and lymphoblasts, all of which are larger than the neutrophil seen in the mid to lower center of the slide. There are multiple small nucleoli in some nuclei, and there is moderate to lightly basophilic cytoplasm. This is compatible with lymphoblastic lymphosarcoma, a high-grade tumor.

Figure 7.40 shows a canine splenic lymphosarcoma biopsy. The normal splenic architecture in this 10-year-old spayed female Maltese dog is replaced by sheets of large lymphocytes and lymphoblasts with scattered macrophages. There were 6 to 12 mitotic figures/HPF, which suggests that this is an aggressive tumor type.

Mast cell tumor

Figure 7.41 shows a feline splenic mastocytosis FNA. This dense population of mast cells was aspirated from an adult neutered male Domestic Shorthair cat with marked splenomegaly and is diagnostic for splenic mast cell tumor. These cells can degranulate, releasing histamine and other vasoactive amines, causing a hypotensive crisis. Large spleens

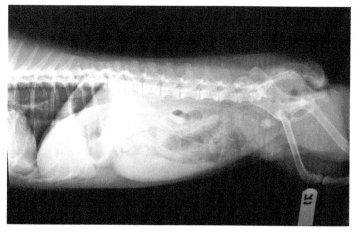

Figure 7.33 Radiograph of a dog with splenomegaly. (Radiograph courtesy of Dr. Laura Hokett.)

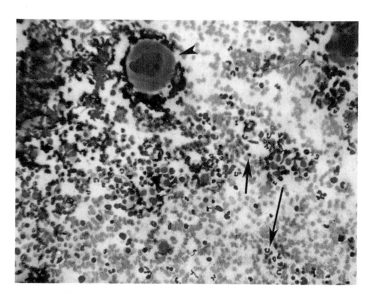

Figure 7.34 Extramedullary hematopoiesis FNA. 10x.

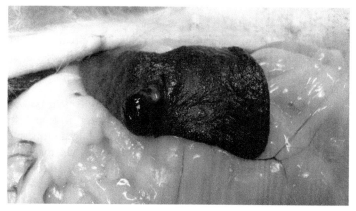

Figure 7.35 Gross picture of a splenic nodule.

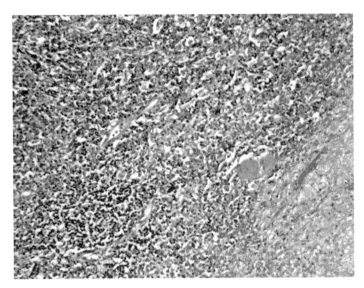

Figure 7.36 Splenic fibrohistiocytic nodule biopsy. 10x.

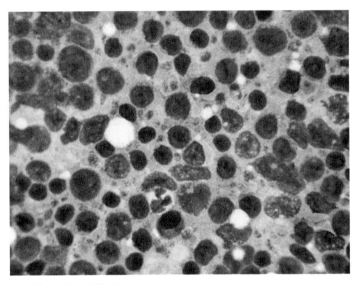

Figure 7.37 Splenic reactive lymphoid hyperplasia FNA. 50x.

should be handled with care prior to removal. Perform a CBC to check for circulating mast cells, and check for skin masses or other enlarged internal organs. Note that many of the neoplastic cells do not appear to have cytoplasmic granules. This is typical of feline mast cells that often are poorly granular on cytologic preparation and might be confused for lymphocytes or macrophages.

Figure 7.42 shows a biopsy of a feline splenic mastocytosis. An enlarged splenic mass was found on ultrasound in a 12-year-old Domestic Medium Hair cat. The patient expired prior to treatment, and a necropsy was performed. A touch preparation from the spleen yielded mast cells. The lymphoid nodules in this spleen were small and widely spaced. The parenchyma is diffusely infiltrated by somewhat enlarged mast cells that are accompanied by scattered eosinophils. Mitotic figures were not seen in the mast cell population after a moderate search. In cats with mastocytosis the infiltrates can be confined to the spleen, in which case splenectomy is the treatment of choice. However, cats with splenic mastocytosis may also have mast cell tumors and mast cell infiltrates in other organs including skin, lymph nodes, and the intestinal tract.

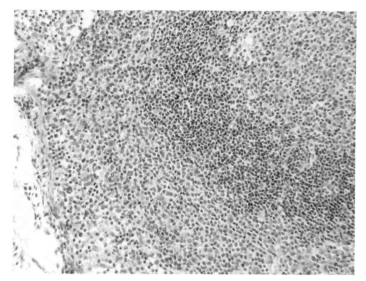

Figure 7.38 Splenic lymphoid nodular hyperplasia biopsy. 10x.

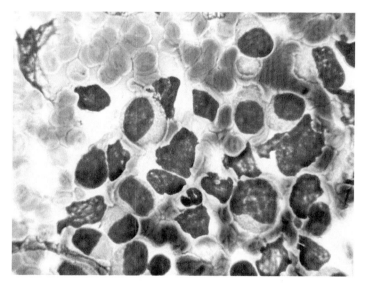

Figure 7.39 Splenic lymphosarcoma FNA. 50x.

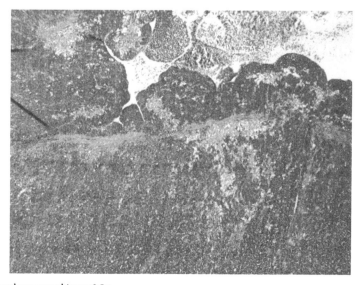

Figure 7.40 Canine splenic lymphosarcoma biopsy. 2.5x.

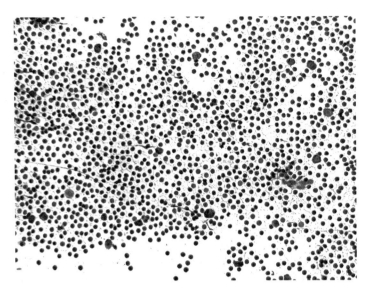

Figure 7.41 Feline splenic mastocytosis FNA. 10x.

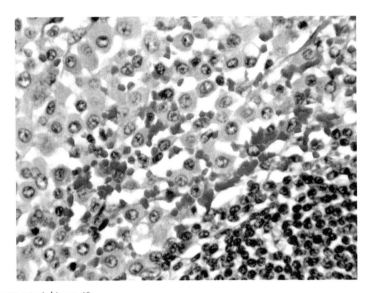

Figure 7.42 Feline splenic mastocytosis biopsy. 40x.

Figure 7.43 shows a biopsy of a feline splenic mast cell tumor. After the FNA of an enlarged spleen in this adult spayed female Domestic Shorthair cat revealed mastocytosis, with a tentative diagnosis of mast cell tumor, the spleen was gently removed surgically and the diagnosis confirmed histologically. Note that the entire splenic parenchyma is packed full of mast cells. Degranulation due to firm palpation or rough handling during surgery has been known to result in fatal hypotension.

Splenic torsion

Figure 7.44 shows a left lateral radiograph of an adult neutered male Bassett Hound dog with splenomegaly.

Figure 7.45 shows an ultrasound of an enlarged spleen resulting from splenic torsion around the splenic artery in the dog shown in Figure 7.44.

Figure 7.46 shows an FNA of canine splenic necrosis. Aspiration of the spleen of the Bassett Hound from Figure 7.44 revealed blood, platelet clumps, and variably necrotic neutrophils with free nuclei from ruptured cells, suggesting necrosis. A laparotomy was performed, resulting in discovery of a splenic torsion.

Figure 7.47 shows a biopsy of canine splenic necrosis. This is a biopsy of the torsed spleen from Figures 7.44 through 7.46. There is diffuse necrosis and scattered areas of hemorrhage with infiltrates of neutrophils at the interface, similar to the population seen on FNA.

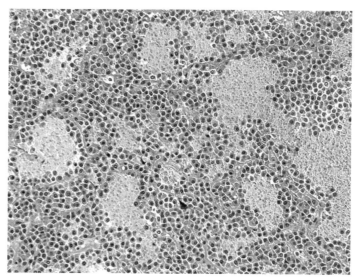

Figure 7.43 Feline splenic mast cell tumor biopsy. 10x.

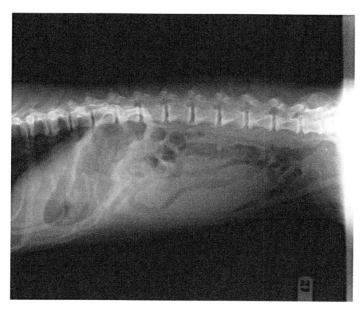

Figure 7.44 Left lateral radiograph of an adult neutered male Bassett Hound dog with splenomegaly. (Radiograph courtesy of Dr. Laura Hokett.)

Splenic hematoma

Figure 7.48 shows an ultrasound of a canine splenic cavitated mass.

Figure 7.49 shows a gross presentation of a cavitated canine splenic mass. Representative sections for histology should be collected at the interface of the necrotic tissue and surrounding normal tissue (arrow).

Figure 7.50 shows an FNA of a canine splenic hematoma. Aspiration of a splenic hematoma may yield a few spindloid to epithelioid cells with small monomorphic nuclei in variably dense blood, neutrophils, and necrotic debris. The strands of oblong nuclei may be from deteriorating blood vessels in areas of necrosis. This can also be seen with hematoma and hemangiosarcoma and is not a distinguishing diagnostic feature. Aspiration of focal cavitated masses is not generally recommended due to the low potential for definitive diagnosis and the high potential for rupture of the mass and intra-abdominal hemorrhage or seeding of neoplastic cells.

Figure 7.51 shows a biopsy of a canine splenic hematoma. A 10-year-old spayed female Golden Retriever presented with splenomegaly. Splenectomy and histologic evaluation revealed a thrombosed large vessel with variably dense infiltrates of neutrophils and heme-laden macrophages in adjacent congested and necrotic stroma, compatible with splenic hematoma formation. The causes of hematoma include traumatic injury, vascular thrombosis or vascular rupture, and extravasation from a vascular tumor not captured on the sections examined.

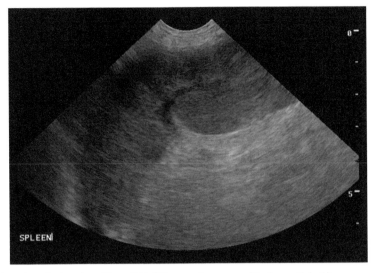

Figure 7.45 Ultrasound of the enlarged spleen from Figure 7.44. (Ultrasound courtesy of Dr. Laura Hokett.)

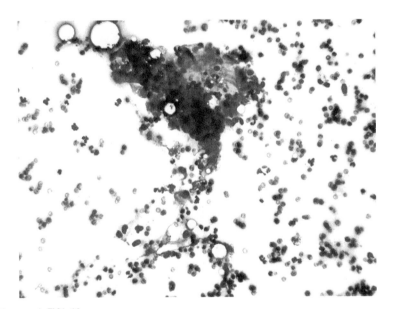

Figure 7.46 Canine splenic necrosis FNA. 10x.

Splenic hemangiosarcoma

Figure 7.52 shows an FNA from a canine splenic hemangiosaroma. Aspiration of an aggressive and proliferative vascular tumor may yield occasional large cells with large nuclei, large nucleoli, and basophilic cytoplasm (arrows). Finding of even low numbers of these cells is suggestive of hemangiosarcoma. This sample was collected postmortem from an adult male Weimaraner that was euthanized due to severe splenomegaly and free abdominal blood. Hemangiosarcoma was histologically confirmed.

Figure 7.53 shows a canine splenic hemangiosarcoma biopsy. A neutered male Golden Retriever of unknown age was presented with lethargy and was diagnosed with hemo-abdomen. Exploratory celiotomy confirmed hemorrhage from a 5-cm-diameter mid splenic mass. No evidence of metastatic disease was seen in the abdomen or on thoracic radiographs. Selected splenic tissue was submitted in formalin. The mass is composed of pleomorphic medium to large round and polygonal vascular endothelial cells with considerable variation in cell and nuclear size. These cells line anastomosing capillary and more cavernous blood-filled spaces in one to multiple layers. Mitoses were seen in this cell population at a rate of 0–3/HPF, and some cells have more than one nucleus. Abnormal mitotic spindles were also noted. These

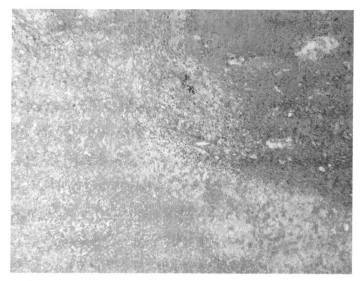

Figure 7.47 Canine splenic necrosis biopsy. 10x.

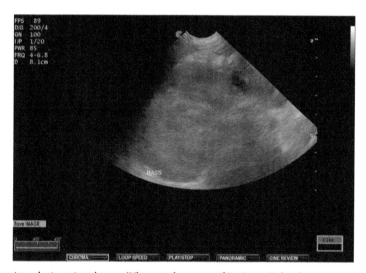

Figure 7.48 Ultrasound of a canine splenic cavitated mass. (Ultrasound courtesy of Dr. Laura Hokett.)

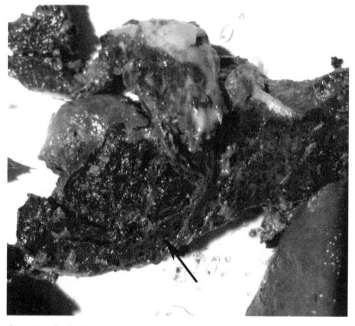

Figure 7.49 Gross photograph of a cavitated splenic mass.

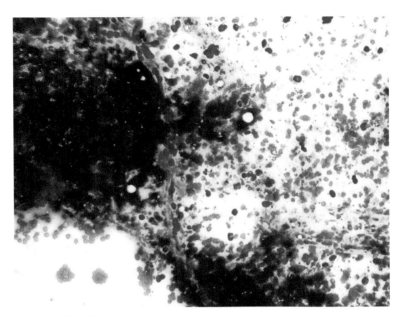

Figure 7.50 Canine splenic hematoma FNA. 10x.

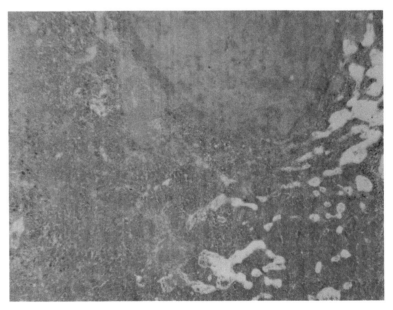

Figure 7.51 Canine splenic hematoma biopsy. 10x.

tumors may be multicentric in the spleen by the time they are discovered. They can metastasize via both blood vessels and lymphatics, and they can also seed the abdomen. Prognosis for long-term survival was considered to be guarded.

Splenic histiocytic sarcoma

Figure 7.54 shows FNA of a canine splenic histiocytic sarcoma. This population of epithelioid cells aspirated from a splenic mass in an adult female mixed breed dog exhibits moderate anisokaryosis and amphophilic cytoplasm. The neoplastic cells often consume erythrocytes (arrows) and cellular debris, and they are sometimes multinucleate. The cells are of histiocytic lineage. When multinucleate, they must be differentiated from megakaryocytes, which have a more granular cytoplasm and multilobular nuclei. Megakaryocytes would not be expected to be seen in large groups in the spleen nor would they exhibit the phagocytic tendency that can be seen in some histiocytic sarcomas or the occasional spindloid appearance.

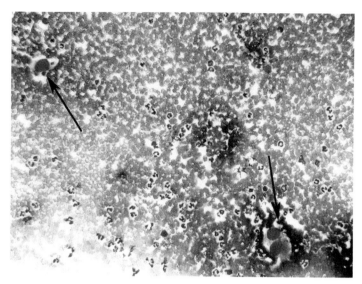

Figure 7.52 Canine splenic hemangiosarcoma FNA. 10x.

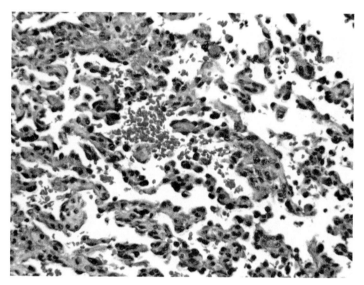

Figure 7.53 Canine splenic hemangiosarcoma biopsy. 20x.

Figure 7.55 shows a canine histocytic sarcoma biopsy. A splenic mass was found in a neutered male 7-year-old Golden Retriever. There is no normal splenic parenchyma in the section. Ischemic necrosis was multifocal. In viable areas the mass is composed of pleomorphic polygonal cells that appear histiocytic. There is considerable variation in cell and nuclear size. The nuclei have one to four nucleoli and a moderate amount of eosinophilic cytoplasm. Cells with double or multiple nuclei are easily found. MI = 13/10 HPF, and abnormal mitotic spindles are present. There is an increased incidence of abnormal histiocytic proliferations in this breed. The lesions may be localized or disseminated. Skin, sub-cutis, liver, spleen, bone marrow, and other sites may be involved as individual tumors or part of a multicentric disease.

Splenic malignant fibrous histiocytoma

Figure 7.56 shows a canine splenic spindle cell tumor FNA. Small clusters of spindle cells can occasionally be seen in normal spleen aspirates, but these large clusters were scattered throughout the sample aspirated from the spleen of a 14-year-old neutered male mixed breed dog with a splenic mass. The cells are well differentiated, with small ovoid to round nuclei, fine chromatin, and pale wispy cytoplasm, but the presence of such high numbers of this cell type is com-patible with spindle cell neoplasia. Biopsy would be necessary for definitive diagnosis.

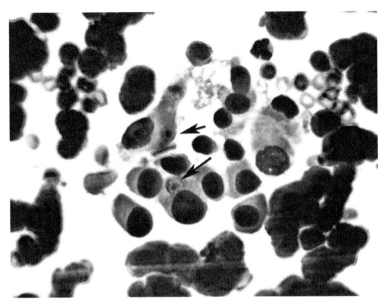

Figure 7.54 Canine splenic histiocytic sarcoma FNA. 50x.

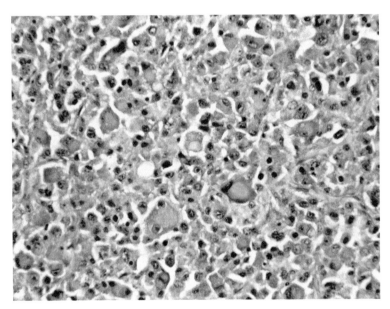

Figure 7.55 Canine histiocytic sarcoma biopsy. 20x.

Figure 7.57 shows a biopsy of a canine splenic malignant fibrous histiocytoma. A splenic mass was seen on a radiograph of a 7-year-old spayed female Pit Bull Terrier with a PCV of 18% at presentation. Abdominal exploratory revealed a 20-cm-diameter round mass in the mid body of the spleen. Two 4-cm-thick slices of spleen with portions of a multinodular very firm white mass each 9.5 cm in greatest dimension were submitted. The mass is composed of large polygonal cells that appear histiocytic. The mass has a moderate collagenous stroma, and it is composed of intersecting fascicles of pleomorphic polygonal and plump spindloid cells that sometimes appear histiocytic and in other areas appear fibroblastic. There is considerable variation in cell and nuclear size. Scattered tumor giant cells were present. Mitoses were seen at a rate of 0–3/HPF depending on area. This splenic mass is most consistent with a malignant fibrous histiocytoma. It is a mixture of the storiform-pleomorphic and inflammatory types. These tumors can be primary in the canine skin and subcutis, or in the spleen. Timely splenectomy is the recommended treatment for tumors in the spleen. However, these tumors can metastasize, and they are sometimes multicentric by the time they are discovered.

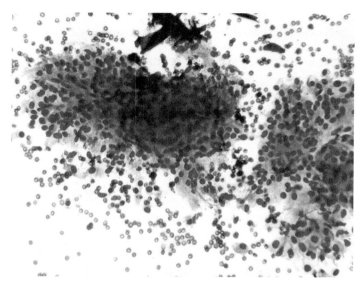

Figure 7.56 Canine splenic spindle cell tumor FNA. 10x.

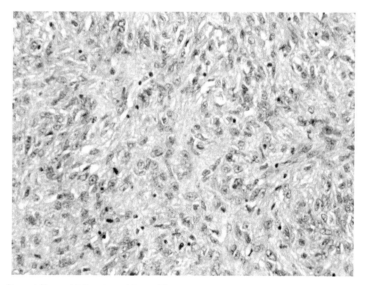

Figure 7.57 Canine splenic malignant fibrous histiocytoma biopsy. 20x.

Additional reading

Diseases that result in liver enlargement

Arndt TP, Shelly SM. The Liver. In Cowell and Tyler's Diagnostic Cytology and Hematology of the Dog and Cat. 4th ed. Valenciano and Cowell. 2014. 354–371.

Cullen JM, Stalker MJ. Liver and Biliary System. In Jubb, Kennedy and Palmer's Pathology of Domestic Animals. Vol 2. 6th ed. M. Grant Maxie, Editor. Elsevier. St Louis. 2016. 258–352.

Liptak, JM. Hepatobiliary Tumors. In Small Animal Clinical Oncology, 5th ed. Withrow and MacEwen. 2013. Elsevier. St. Louis. 405–412.

Meyer DJ. The Liver. In Canine and Feline Cytology; A Color Atlas and Interpretation Guide. 3rd ed. Raskin and Meyer. 2016. Elsevier. St. Louis. 259–283.

Vacuolar hepatopathy

Center SA. Hepatic Lipidosis. In Blackwell's Five-Minute Veterinary Consult: Canine and Feline. 5th ed. Tilley LP and Smith FWK, Jr. 2011. John Wiley & Sons, Inc. West Sussex, UK. 560–561.

Center SA. Vacuolar Hepatopathy. In Blackwell's Five-Minute Veterinary Consult: Canine and Feline. 5th ed. Tilley LP and Smith FWK, Jr. 2011. John Wiley & Sons, Inc. West Sussex, UK. 1286–87.

Nodular regeneration with bile duct hyperplasia

Center SA. Hepatic Nodular Hyperplasia. In Blackwell's Five-Minute Veterinary Consult: Canine and Feline. 5th ed. Tilley LP and Smith FWK, Jr. 2011. John Wiley & Sons, Inc. West Sussex, UK. 562.

Hepatocellular neoplasia

Morrison WB. Hepatocellular Adenoma. In Blackwell's Five-Minute Veterinary Consult: Canine and Feline. 5th ed. Tilley LP and Smith FWK, Jr. 2011. John Wiley & Sons, Inc. West Sussex, UK. 572.

Morrison WB. Hepatocellular Carcinoma. In Blackwell's Five-Minute Veterinary Consult: Canine and Feline. 5th ed. Tilley LP and Smith FWK, Jr. 2011. John Wiley & Sons, Inc. West Sussex, UK. 573.

Bile duct carcinoma

Clifford C. Bile Duct Carcinoma. In Blackwell's Five-Minute Veterinary Consult: Canine and Feline. 5th ed. Tilley LP and Smith FWK, Jr. 2011. John Wiley & Sons, Inc. West Sussex, UK. 168.

Hepatic hemangiosarcoma

Clifford C. Hemangiosarcoma, Spleen and Liver. In Blackwell's Five-Minute Veterinary Consult: Canine and Feline. 5th ed. Tilley LP and Smith FWK, Jr. 2011. John Wiley & Sons, Inc. West Sussex, UK. 545–546.

Lymphoma

Keller SM, Vernau W, Hodges J, et al. Hepatosplenic and Hepatocytotopic T-Cell Lymphoma: Two Distinct Types of T-Cell Lymphoma in Dogs. Vet Path 2012; 50:281–290.

Gastrointestinal lesions

Haddad JL, Marks Stowe DA, Neel JA. The Gastrointestinal Tract. In Cowell and Tyler's Diagnostic Cytology and Hematology of the Dog and Cat. 4th ed. Valenciano and Cowell. 2014. 312–340.

Jergens AE, Jones Hostetter S, Andreasen CB. Oral Cavity, Gastrointestinal Tract, and Associated Structures. In Canine and Feline Cytology; A Color Atlas and Interpretation Guide. 3rd ed. Raskin and Meyer. 2016. Elsevier. St. Louis. 220–246.

Selting KA. Intestinal Tumors. In Small Animal Clinical Oncology, 5th ed. Withrow and MacEwen. 2013. Elsevier. St. Louis. 412–431.

Uzal FA, Plattner BL, Hostetter JM. Alimentary System. In Jubb, Kennedy, and Palmer's Pathology of Domestic Animals. Vol 2. 6th ed. M. Grant Maxie, Editor. Elsevier. St Louis. 2016. 1–258.

Eosinophilic inflammatory bowel disease
Lymphoplasmacellular inflammatory bowel disease

Jergens AE. Inflammatory Bowel Disease. In Blackwell's Five-Minute Veterinary Consult: Canine and Feline. 5th ed. Tilley LP and Smith FWK, Jr. 2011. John Wiley & Sons, Inc. West Sussex, UK. 700–701.

Gastrointestinal malignant lymphoma

Coyle KA, Steinberg H. Characterization of Lymphocytes in Canine Gastrointestinal Lymphoma. Vet Path 2004; 41:141–146.

Gastrointestinal adenocarcinoma

Garrett LD. Adenocarcinoma, Stomach, Small and Large Intestine, Rectal. In Blackwell's Five-Minute Veterinary Consult: Canine and Feline. 5th ed. Tilley LP and Smith FWK, Jr. 2011. John Wiley & Sons, Inc. West Sussex, UK. 32.

Gastrointestinal spindle cell tumor

Garrett LD. Leiomyoma, Stomach, Small and Large Intestine. In Blackwell's Five-Minute Veterinary Consult: Canine and Feline. 5th ed. Tilley LP and Smith FWK, Jr. 2011. John Wiley & Sons, Inc. West Sussex, UK. 741.

Garrett LD. Leiomyosarcoma, Stomach, Small and Large Intestine. In Blackwell's Five-Minute Veterinary Consult: Canine and Feline. 5th ed. Tilley LP and Smith FWK, Jr. 2011. John Wiley & Sons, Inc. West Sussex, UK. 742.

Kidney and bladder masses

Borjesson DL, DeJong K. Urinary Tract. In Canine and Feline Cytology; A Color Atlas and Interpretation Guide. 3rd ed. Raskin and Meyer. 2016. Elsevier. St. Louis. 284–294.

Cianciolo RE, Mohr FC. Urinary System. In Jubb, Kennedy, and Palmer's Pathology of Domestic Animals. Vol 2. 6th ed. M. Grant Maxie, Editor. Elsevier. St Louis. 2016. 376–464.

Ewing PJ, Meinkoth JH, Cowell RL, Tyler RD. The Kidneys. In Cowell and Tyler's Diagnostic Cytology and Hematology of the Dog and Cat. 4th ed. Valenciano and Cowell. 2014. 387–401.

Pyogranulomatous inflammatory disease suggestive of feline infectious peritonitis
Scott FW. Feline Infectious Peritonitis. In Blackwell's Five-Minute Veterinary Consult: Canine and Feline. 5th ed. Tilley LP and Smith FWK, Jr. 2011. John Wiley & Sons, Inc. West Sussex, UK. 468–469.

Renal carcinoma
Chun R. Adenocarcinoma, Renal. In Blackwell's Five-Minute Veterinary Consult: Canine and Feline. 5th ed. Tilley LP and Smith FWK, Jr. 2011. John Wiley & Sons, Inc. West Sussex, UK. 29.

Urinary bladder cystitis with reactive epithelial hyperplasia
Urinary bladder polyp
Osborne CA, Lulich JP. Polypoid Cystitis. In Blackwell's Five-Minute Veterinary Consult: Canine and Feline. 5th ed. Tilley LP and Smith FWK, Jr. 2011. John Wiley & Sons, Inc. West Sussex, UK. 1028–1029.

Transitional cell carcinoma
Chun R. Transitional Cell Carcinoma. In Blackwell's Five-Minute Veterinary Consult: Canine and Feline. 5th ed. Tilley LP and Smith FWK, Jr. 2011. John Wiley & Sons, Inc. West Sussex, UK. 1247–1248.

Knapp DW, McMillan SK. Tumors of the Urinary System. In Small Animal Clinical Oncology, 5th ed. Withrow and MacEwen. 2013. Elsevier. St. Louis. 572–582.

Splenomegaly and splenic masses

Raskin RE. Hemolymphatic System. In Canine and Feline Cytology; A Color Atlas and Interpretation Guide. 3rd ed. Raskin and Meyer. 2016. Elsevier. St. Louis. 91–137.

MacWilliams PS, McManus PM. The Spleen. In Cowell and Tyler's Diagnostic Cytology and Hematology of the Dog and Cat. 4th ed. Valenciano and Cowell. 2014. 372–386.

Valli VEO, Kiupel M, Bienzle D. Hematopoietic System. In Jubb, Kennedy and Palmer's Pathology of Domestic Animals. Vol 3. 6th ed. M. Grant Maxie, Editor. Elsevier. St Louis. 2016. 102–268.

Extramedullary hematopoiesis
Balkman CE. Splenomegaly. In Blackwell's Five-Minute Veterinary Consult: Canine and Feline. 5th ed. Tilley LP and Smith FWK, Jr. 2011. John Wiley & Sons, Inc. West Sussex, UK. 1179–1180.

Lymphoid nodular hyperplasia
Spangler WL, Kass PH. Pathologic and prognostic characteristics of splenomegaly in dogs due to fibrohistiocytic nodules: 98 cases. Vet Path 1998; 35:488–498.

Mast cell tumor
London CA, Thamm DH. Mast Cell Tumors. In Small Animal Clinical Oncology, 5th ed. Withrow and MacEwen. 2013. Elsevier. St. Louis. 335–355.

Splenic torsion

Rozanski EA. Splenic Torsion. In Blackwell's Five-Minute Veterinary Consult: Canine and Feline. 5th ed. Tilley LP and Smith FWK, Jr. 2011. John Wiley & Sons, Inc. West Sussex, UK. 1178.

Splenic hemangiosarcoma

Clifford C. Hemangiosarcoma, Spleen and Liver. In Blackwell's Five-Minute Veterinary Consult: Canine and Feline. 5th ed. Tilley LP and Smith FWK, Jr. 2011. John Wiley & Sons, Inc. West Sussex, UK. 545–546.

Thamm DH. Hemangiosarcoma. In Small Animal Clinical Oncology, 5th ed. Withrow and MacEwen. 2013. Elsevier. St. Louis. 679–688.

8 Sample Handling

This final chapter offers suggestions for obtaining the best possible results from a cytologic or biopsy sample. It is a source of frustration and lost opportunity when a sample is invalidated by inappropriate collection or inadequate processing.

Cytologic specimens

Cytology samples can be collected by impressing the slide to a lesion or by placing a small drop of fluid on a slide and laying another slide over it and gently drawing the slides over each other. The techniques for collecting samples and making slides are well illustrated in many cytology texts. Figures 8.1 to 8.3 are examples of slides received at a commercial laboratory. A good preparation technique results in a preparation that will have thin areas, some thick areas, and edges that do not extend to the sides of the slide (Figure 8.1). This type of preparation is made by placing the flat surface of two slides together and sliding them apart. The sliding apart step should happen quickly or the sample layer between the slides may spread out and become thin with rupture of the cells. If the slides dry together the protein in the sample will act like a glue, and the slides will become inseparable, making it impossible to stain them. Unless the slide is marked at the point of care with a label, use only frosted edge slides for cytology preparations so they can be labeled with pencil or indelible marker. Only diamond etching will permanently mark shiny glass, as all other markers can wash off in the alcohol phase of staining (Figure 8.2), leaving the identification illegible. Slides with large amounts of sample (Figure 8.3) will have few areas of good cellular detail. The stain may not penetrate the thicker areas where the cells will be piled on each other, diagnostic cells may be trapped at the edge of the slide where the stage of the microscope may interfere with the focus, or part of the sample may be covered by a label. From a medicolegal point of view, there is no assurance that a slide without the clinician's identifying information (at least a patient name) is the correct sample. Writing the information on the slide holder without identifying the slides is not adequate, because the slides can be removed from the holder and marked incorrectly.

Cytologic preparations to be stained with Wright-Giemsa (W-G) stain should be fixed in methanol. Unfixed cytology slides should not be refrigerated, as the condensation of moisture on the slide surface can rupture the cells (Figure 8.4). Unfixed slides should not be shipped to a laboratory in the same box as biopsy samples, as this can result in exposure to formalin vapors that will make the cells refractory to staining with W-G stain (Figure 8.5). Fixation in methanol prior to shipping will prevent these common artifacts. The fixative should be refreshed frequently, because old and depleted fixative can produce artifacts such as loss of cells from the slide, failure to stain, refractile bubbles in the cells, and in the case of mast cells, elution of mast cell granules during the aqueous phase of staining.

The most common cytologic stain is modified W-G stain (also known as quick dip stain) (Figure 8.6), which will stain cells, bacteria, fungi, parasites, and various artifacts, but it will not stain crystals or *Mycobacteria*.

Depleted stain can result in artifacts that make accurate cytologic evaluation difficult. Usually the basophilic component fails to penetrate the nucleus of the cells so diagnostic nuclear changes can be missed. Inadequately stained slides can sometimes be decolorized with methanol fixative and restained. Overstained slides can occasionally be salvaged in this manner but usually the stain remains too dense for accurate evaluation. Acceptable stain quality clearly differentiates the nucleus from the cytoplasm with sharp margins and good contrast. It is possible to identify slides that are

---

Atlas for the Diagnosis of Tumors in the Dog and Cat, First Edition. Anita R. Kiehl and Maron Brown Calderwood Mays.
© 2016 John Wiley & Sons, Inc. Published 2016 by John Wiley & Sons, Inc.

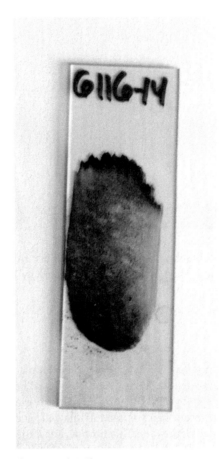

Figure 8.1 Well-made cytology preparation. Wright-Giemsa (W-G).

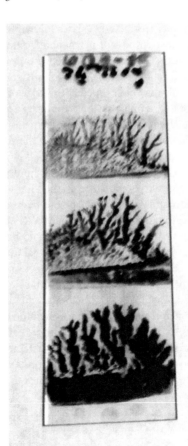

Figure 8.2 Illegible identifying marks on a non-frosted slide. W-G.

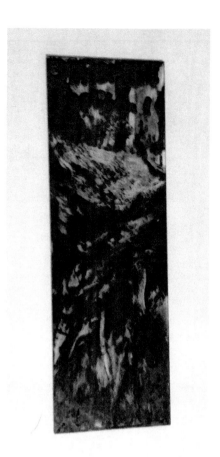

Figure 8.3 Poorly made cytology preparation. W-G.

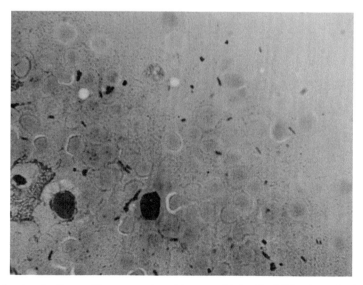

Figure 8.4 A 40-power view of ruptured cells caused by exposure to moisture on a dried unfixed slide prior to fixation. W-G.

under-stained by gross observation. A series of eight slides was submitted with four already stained by the referring clinic (Figure 8.7). The four slides stained dark blue stain (arrow) are typical of adequate stain quality, and cells on these slides will have good nuclear and cytoplasmic detail (Figure 8.8). The four slides stained light pink with splotches of blue (arrowhead) are typical of inadequate stain quality and will have poor nuclear and cytoplasmic detail (Figure 8.9).

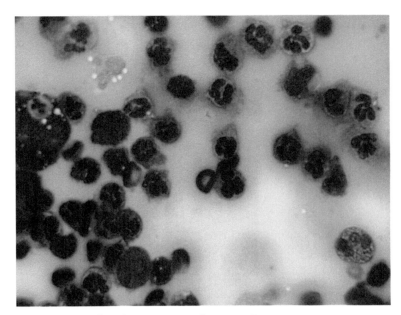

Figure 8.5 A 50-power view of cells exposed to formalin vapors prior to fixation. W-G.

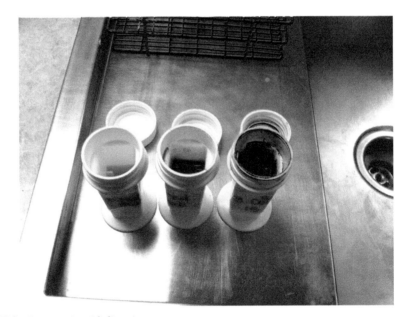

Figure 8.6 Modified Wright-Giemsa stain quick dip stain set up.

Identification of poorly stained slides by gross examination will allow additional stain time to be added before the use of a cover-slip or immersion oil, either of which will prevent further staining.

Wet preps made with aqueous new methylene blue (NMB) are only viable for a few hours, because the cells will degenerate over time even if the wet prep is preserved with a sealant (Figure 8.10, Figure 8.11). If a wet prep is prepared for point of care preliminary diagnosis, some sample should be set aside, or smears made, before adding the stain to the wet sample. Once the wet stain is introduced to the sample, additional staining with Wright-Giemsa is generally unsuccessful.

Ultrasound gel and lubricant will stain dark purple to magenta. This should be kept in mind when collecting samples (Figure 8.12), because this material can be dragged into the sample by a needle or catheter, and can mask cells and bacteria when present in dense clumps.

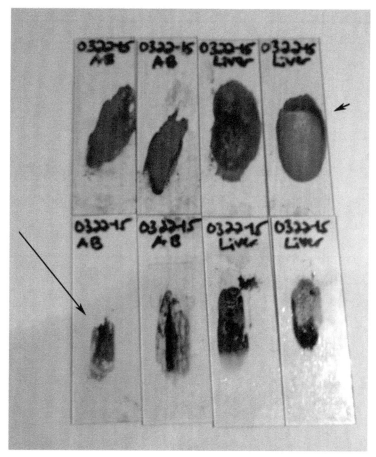

Figure 8.7 Gross comparison of well-stained (dark blue) slides versus poorly stained (brown) slides. W-G.

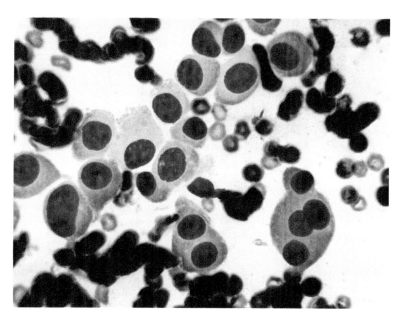

Figure 8.8 Well-stained cytologic preparation viewed on 40 power. W-G.

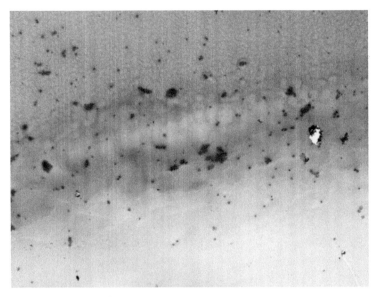

Figure 8.9 Understained cytologic preparation viewed on 40 power. W-G.

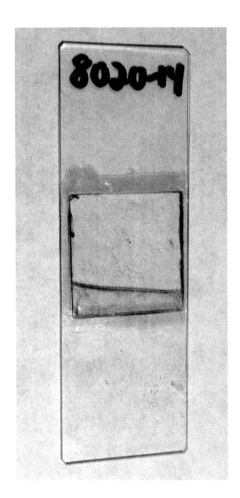

Figure 8.10 New Methylene Blue wet prep.

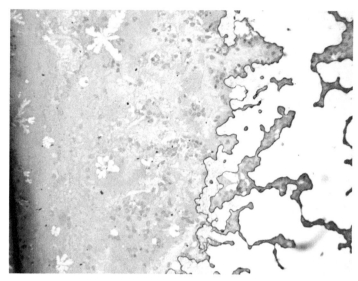

Figure 8.11 High-power evaluation of an aged wet prep.

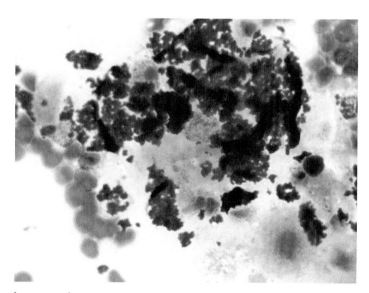

Figure 8.12 Ultrasound gel artifact on a cytologic preparation. W-G.

Biopsy specimens

Biopsy samples will exhibit optimum cellular detail if placed immediately after collection into 10% buffered neutral formalin. If samples are not placed in formalin within a few hours they will begin to autolyze and the cells will lose their integrity and form.

Biopsy containers should be plastic wide neck jars with screw tops (Figure 8.13), not glass or narrow neck jars (Figure 8.14, Figure 8.15, Figure 8.16) or pop-top plastic food containers (Figure 8.17). If a large sample must be folded or forced into a narrow-mouthed jar, once it is fixed it will be difficult to remove from the jar without cutting it into pieces and destroying the margins, or breaking the jar (Figure 8.15). Adhesive tape is not recommended to hold a lid in place, because it is not waterproof and will not prevent leakage, and it will make it difficult to remove the top. A common cause of leakage during transport is cross threading of the lid caused by failure to seat the lid properly. This typically causes loss of formalin into the bag and absorbent material, and sometimes results in the loss of tiny samples such as needle or endoscopic biopsies.

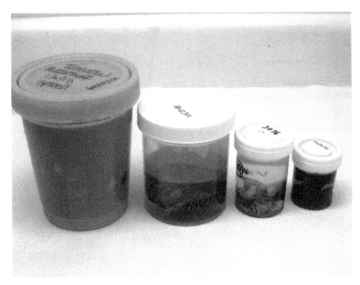

Figure 8.13 Acceptable jars for submission of specimens for histology.

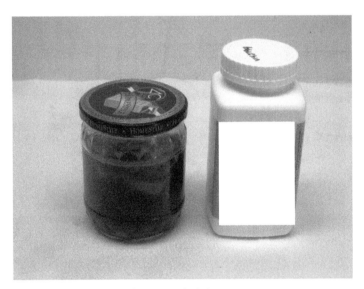

Figure 8.14 Unacceptable specimen jars include glass jars and narrow necked plastic jars.

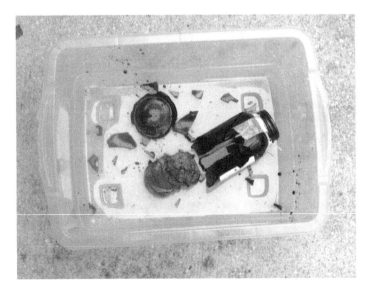

Figure 8.15 Broken glass jar.

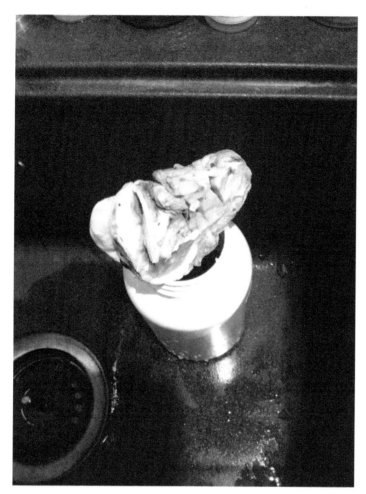

Figure 8.16 A large testicle was presented in this narrow neck plastic jar.

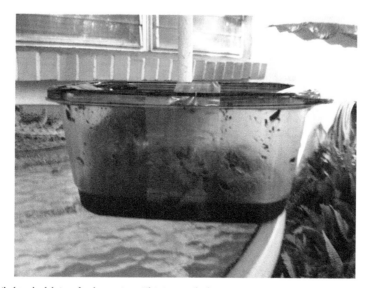

Figure 8.17 Large spleen mailed to the lab in a food container. This is not a leak-resistant container. Note that there is very little formalin remaining in the container.

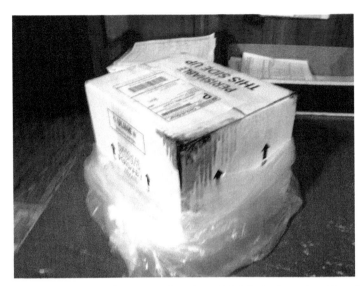

Figure 8.18 This formalin-soaked outer box contained the specimen from Figure 8.17. It had to be retrieved from the courier who refused to deliver it.

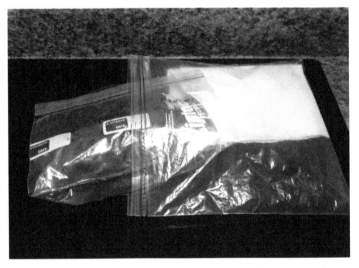

Figure 8.19 Large samples may be submitted in appropriately prepared sealed bags. (See text for instruction.)

A sample that is too large to fit into a plastic screw top jar can be placed in a strong sealable plastic bag. That bag is then wrapped in absorbent materials and placed in another larger sealable bag that is then placed in a hard shippable container that can protect the bags and prevent formalin from leaking out if there is a breach in the bags. Formalin leaking from a package during shipping is considered biohazardous and may result in a fine, disposal of the sample as hazardous waste by the courier, and a resultant hazardous waste charge made to the shipper (Figure 8.18). If this is a sample that is to be sent through commercial service to a distant site it would be prudent to fix the sample in 10% buffered neutral formalin then pour off the excess formalin prior to shipping (Figure 8.19).

Small samples that fit in a 60-ml biopsy jar can usually be sent using a standard biopsy protocol. The carrier should be contacted for instructions when shipping samples in formalin, including the maximum amount of formalin allowed, the type of outer packaging, and instructions for outer labeling. 10% buffered neutral formalin less than a certain amount, (usually 35 ml), is generally not considered to be biohazardous as long as it is contained appropriately. Most instructions require a primary screw top plastic container surrounded by absorbent material within a secondary sealable bag, within a tertiary sturdy box (Figure 8.20). Some require an outer plastic bag as well.

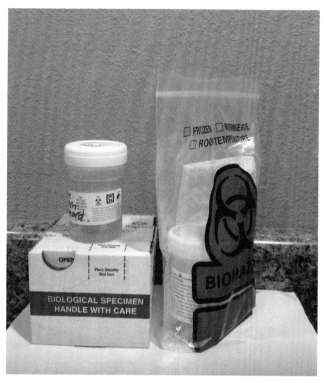

Figure 8.20 A specimen for histology ideally will fit into a screw-top sturdy plastic container that is placed in a pinch-top bag containing absorbent material. The paperwork is slipped into an outer pocket on the bag, and the bag is placed in a firm box.

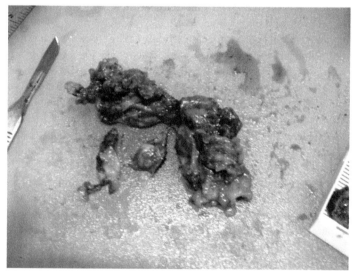

Figure 8.21 Sectioning of unfixed tissue can result in fragmentation of the tissue.

The lab request should be in an outer pocket of the secondary bag so it does not get soaked in formalin if there is a leak. The sample should be marked "Diagnostic specimen," and a return address must be provided. The fines for violations of the federal hazardous material transportation law can be $250 to $27,500 for each violation, and the shipper is the responsible party. Subsequent pickups can be refused.

Small samples should be fixed prior to cutting in order to avoid shredding the tissue (Figure 8.21). Large masses such as a spleen can be cut into smaller portions and identified as to location on the container. If a skin mass is submitted, a cut can be made in the surface of the skin to allow fixation of the center of the tissue, but caution is advised if cutting into the deep margin because any tearing or shredding makes it difficult to confirm that there is normal tissue at all aspects of the deep margin. If a cut is made in the deep margin, tissue shrinkage during fixation can result in exposure of the tumor as the underlying fascia pulls back and this gives a false appearance of tumor extending to the deep margin. Try to avoid tumor margins when making cuts prior to fixation.

If it is necessary to evaluate a particular margin, the location should be marked with a suture or ink. Multiple sutures or different colored inks can be used for additional sites. Gross margins, the size of the mass, and the number of samples submitted should be recorded in the patient record. If a lesion is removed in many small fragments, the surgical margin must be indicated on each tissue if documentation of complete excision is required.

It is important to submit appropriately completed forms with laboratory samples. If there is not a name, species, breed, sex, location, and description of the lesion, and a brief clinical history, potentially valuable diagnostic information may be lost, and the biopsy report may not be the most comprehensive result possible. If slides are submitted there should be a label directly on each slide. All jars, not just the lids, should be labeled in indelible ink with the patient name and the referring doctor or hospital.

Histology processing, glass slide production, and routine staining

The following is a brief overview of how a biopsy is made into a slide. Fresh or poorly fixed tissues must be fixed in 10% buffered neutral buffered formalin at a ratio of 10 parts fixative to 1 part tissue prior to processing, which can result in delay of a day or more. The use of pure formalin or non-buffered formalin is not advised because it is a strong respiratory irritant and can result in tissue fixation artifacts. Delaying fixing also may result in artifacts due to tissue autolysis.

The containers are assigned numbers for identification of the cases. The specimens are examined grossly, described, margins are measured, and sometimes inked if malignancy is suspected. Specimens are also inked using different colors if there are multiple tissues that must be differentiated as to site. Specimens containing bone are decalcified before tissue processing. A technician or pathologist then cuts small representative sections of the tissues to be examined microscopically and places them in corresponding numbered plastic cassettes. The tissues are then processed, usually in an automatic processor that dehydrates the tissues, clears the tissues of the dehydrants, and infiltrates them with liquid paraffin. Tissue processors usually run for 9 to 12 hours. The tissue sections are then manually embedded in molten paraffin by a technician who properly orients them before the paraffin hardens. When the paraffin blocks are hard, thin sections are cut from the blocks by a technician using a microtome. The thin sections are floated in a warm water bath and picked up on a glass slide. The sections are warmed in an oven for about 15 minutes to help the sections adhere to the slides. The sections must then be deparaffinized. The glass slides with adhered thin tissue sections are stained with hematoxylin and eosin (H&E). The stained slides are cover-slipped, labeled, and reviewed before delivery to the pathologist. Recuts are sometimes necessary if there are wrinkles, tears, or the orientation is not perfect.

The pathologist receives the trays of slides with the case information and formulates the report. There are numerous places where a delay can occur, but there are few places that can be shortened or skipped to decrease turnaround time.

Biopsies are usually stained with hematoxalin and eosin, which stains cells very well but is often less than adequate for bacteria, fungus, some parasites, and cytoplasmic granules in poorly differentiated tumors, such as mast cell granules in pleomorphic high-grade mast cell tumors. Special stains are sometimes requested to look for infectious agents and tumor cell markers. Examples are Brown and Brenn (BB) Gram stain for bacteria, Ziehl-Neelsen and Fite's stains for acid–fast bacteria (Figure 8.22, Figure 8.23), Periodic acid-Schiff (PAS) stain for fungal elements, Gomori methenamine Silver (GMS) stain for fungal elements and Pythium and Lagenidium fragments, and Giemsa and Toluidine Blue stains for mast cell granules (Figure 8.24, Figure 8.25).

A few immunohistochemical stains can be used on formalin-fixed paraffin-embedded tissues. The stains commonly requested in veterinary medicine are anti-CD79a (Figure 8.26, Figure 8.27) and anti-CD20 (depending on availability of the reagent), which are used to identify canine and feline B lymphocytes in malignant lymphoma. Canine and feline T lymphocytes are stained with anti-CD3 (Figure 8.28). Identical serial sections are incubated with buffer only (negative control), as well as with the primary antibody, and then counterstained with hematoxylin. Sometimes spindle cell tumors are stained with anti-S100 to differentiate canine neurofibrosarcomas (positive) from fibrosarcomas (negative), but the results can be disappointing on formalin-fixed tissue sections.

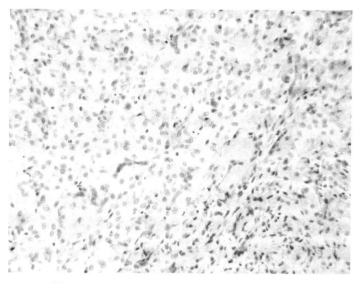

Figure 8.22 Biopsy of a nasal mass in an adult cat showing many epithelioid and multinucleate cells with vaguely granular cytoplasm. H&E. 40x.

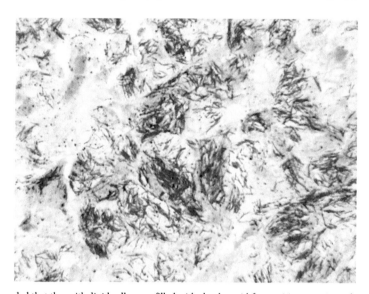

Figure 8.23 Acid fast stain revealed that the epithelioid cells were filled with slender acid fast positive organisms that were identified as a Mycobacteria species by PCR.

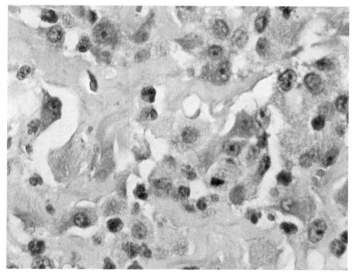

Figure 8.24 Mast cell tumors can sometimes be poorly granular with H&E stain.

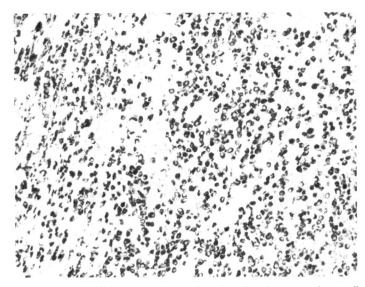

Figure 8.25 Toluidine blue or Giemsa stain can highlight cytoplasmic granules and confirm the suspected mast cell tumor. This technique is especially useful to differentiate between the much more benign histiocytoma that can sometimes mimic mast cell tumor.

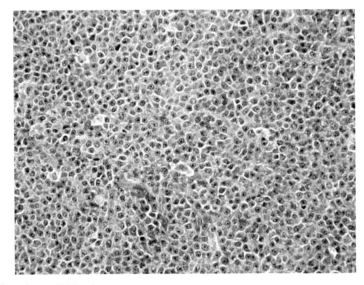

Figure 8.26 Malignant lymphoma biopsy, H&E stain.

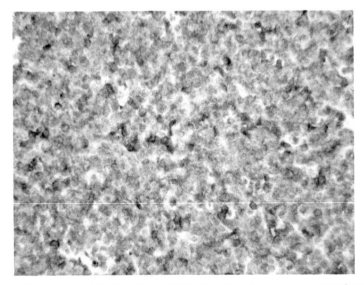

Figure 8.27 Malignant lymphoma biopsy, immunohistochemistry for CD79a. The B lymphocytes present are indicated by the brown stain.

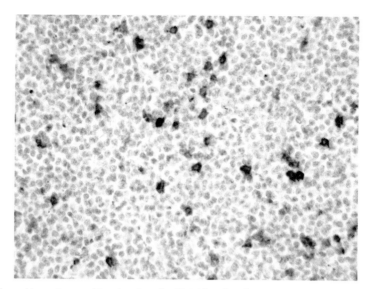

Figure 8.28 Malignant lymphoma biopsy, immunohistochemistry for CD3. The T lymphocytes present are indicated by the dark brown stain.

A few important molecular markers can currently be identified in formalin-fixed, paraffin-embedded veterinary tissues. An example is the frequent evaluation of various key molecules in canine mast cell tumors to help in giving a more accurate prognosis for the patient. These markers include C-Kit, Ki-67, and Agnor (for argyrophilic nuclear organizer regions), among others.

Additional reading

Avery AC, Olver C, Khanna C, Paoloni M. Molecular Diagnostics. In Small Animal Clinical Oncology, 5th ed. Withrow and MacEwen. 2013. Elsevier. St. Louis. 131–142.

Ramos-Vara JA, Avery PR, Avery AC. Advanced Diagnostic Techniques. In Canine and Feline Cytology; A Color Atlas and Interpretation Guide. 3rd ed. Raskin and Meyer. 2016. Elsevier. St. Louis. 453–494.

Cytology specimens

Barger AM. Immunocytochemistry. In Cowell and Tyler's Diagnostic Cytology and Hematology of the Dog and Cat. 4th ed. Valenciano and Cowell. 2014. 532–539.

Corn SC, Chapman SE, Pieczarka EM. Flow Cytometry. In Cowell and Tyler's Diagnostic Cytology and Hematology of the Dog and Cat. 4th ed. Valenciano and Cowell. 2014. 540–549.

Friedrichs KR, Young KM. Diagnostic Cytopathology in Clinical Oncology. In Small Animal Clinical Oncology, 5th ed. Withrow and MacEwen. 2013. Elsevier. St. Louis. 111–130.

Leutenegger CM, Cornwell D. Molecular Methods in Lymphoid Malignancies. In Cowell and Tyler's Diagnostic Cytology and Hematology of the Dog and Cat. 4th ed. Valenciano and Cowell. 2014. 550–553.

Meinkoth JH, Cowell RL, Tyler RD, Morton RJ. Sample Collection and Preparation. In Cowell and Tyler's Diagnostic Cytology and Hematology of the Dog and Cat. 4th ed. Valenciano and Cowell. 2014. 1–19.

Meyer DJ. The Acquisition and Management of Cytology Specimens. In Canine and Feline Cytology; A Color Atlas and Interpretation Guide. 3rd ed. Raskin and Meyer. 2016. Elsevier. St. Louis. 1–15.

Biopsy specimens

Ehrhart NP, Withrow SJ. Biopsy Principles. In Small Animal Clinical Oncology, 5th ed. Withrow and MacEwen. 2013. Elsevier. St. Louis. 143–148.

Farese JP, Withrow SJ. Surgical Oncology. In Small Animal Clinical Oncology, 5th ed. Withrow and MacEwen. 2013. Elsevier. St. Louis. 149–156.

Index

Page numbers ending with f indicate figures and t indicate tables.

Atlas for the Diagnosis of Tumors in the Dog and Cat, First Edition. Anita R. Kiehl and Maron Brown Calderwood Mays.
© 2016 John Wiley & Sons, Inc. Published 2016 by John Wiley & Sons, Inc.

Printed and bound by CPI Group (UK) Ltd, Croydon, CR0 4YY